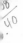

Understanding Stuttering

Berkeley College

From the Library

of

Understanding Health and Sickness Series
Miriam Bloom, Ph.D.
General Editor

Understanding Stuttering

Nathan Lavid, M.D.

University Press of Mississippi
Jackson

www.upress.state.ms.us

The University Press of Mississippi is a member of the Association of American University Presses.

Illustrations by Alan Estridge

11 10 09 08 07 06 05 04 03 4 3 2 1
∞
Library of Congress Cataloging-in-Publication Data

Lavid, Nathan.
Understanding stuttering / Nathan Lavid.
p. ; cm.—(Understanding health and sickness series)
Includes bibliographical references and index.
ISBN 1-57806-572-0 (cloth : alk. paper) —
ISBN 1-57806-573-9 (pbk. : alk. paper)
1. Stuttering [DNLM: 1. Stuttering—physiopathology.
2. Stuttering—therapy. WM 475 L411u 2003] I. Title. II. Series.

RC424.L35 2003
616.85′54—dc21   2002155417

British Library Cataloging-in-Publication Data available

Contents

Acknowledgments

I would like to express my gratitude to the following for making this book a reality. Miriam Bloom, Seetha Srinivasan, Anne Stascavage, and the supportive staff at the University Press of Mississippi, who agreed to tackle this project and provided suggestions that made this book much more readable. Dayana Carcamo, Victoria Dunckley, David Franklin, Louis Gottschalk, Thomas Johnson, Gerald Maguire, Steven Mee, Tony Ortiz, Lawrence Plon, Kenneth Steinhoff, Glyndon Riley, and Joseph Wu, who all composed the stuttering research group while I was in the Department of Psychiatry at the University of California, Irvine, and promoted my understanding of stuttering. Laurence Greenberg, whose criticism and encouragement solidified my thinking about stuttering, such that I was comfortable putting it into words. Sewite Negash at the Pacific Northwest National Laboratory, who kindly assisted in my literature review, patiently answered my queries on basic molecular mechanisms, and tolerated me in general. The two better writers in the Lavid clan, Linda and Brian, who shared their skill—possibly to protect our surname—to make the prose comprehensible to the layperson. Last, the patients I have treated for stuttering over the past few years. They have made this project memorable.

Introduction

The aim of this book is to present stuttering from a medical viewpoint and discuss effective treatment in layman terms. Recent advances reveal that stuttering is a genetic, brain-based condition that can be successfully treated.

The book begins with explanations of how the medical condition of stuttering differs from the stuttering that affects us all. After defining what stuttering is, the population that is affected is presented. How stuttering presents in children, who is more likely to recover, and the associations of acquired stuttering and Tourette syndrome are discussed. Next, basic brain anatomy and function and how the brain processes language are explained. Brain processes that mediate stuttering are presented in relation to when and how they were discovered. In addition, the genetic contribution to stuttering is explored.

Treatment options are presented and explained within this neuroscience framework. The success of these treatments is examined in light of what is known about brain function at the neuronal and molecular level.

The last chapter discusses the most promising cutting-edge research and how the findings of this research will improve treatments and provide a possible cure. The book ends with practical tips on how to converse with those who stutter and a short list of organizations that provide additional information and support for those who stutter.

The focus of this book is one of understanding. A bibliography and glossary are provided to help in this process. All of the resources used during the preparation of this book are listed in the bibliography; the clinical vignettes are based on real patients, but details have been changed to protect confidentiality.

Understanding Stuttering

1. Stuttering Defined

Tongue-Tied

The first step in understanding stuttering is to differentiate the occasional stuttering we all experience from the medical condition of stuttering. Stuttering is a generic term that describes speech that does not follow normal, conventional rhythm. In this sense, we all stutter. When we are speaking too fast, angry, confused, nervous, surprised, or at a loss for words, we get "tongue-tied" and stutter. Over one hundred different muscles in the speech apparatus need to contract or lengthen with some synchronicity to speak without error. This complexity increases when breathing patterns are taken into account. Considering intricacies of speech production, it is expected a mistake will be made from time to time, most commonly when we are angry, confused, speaking too fast, and so on.

Speaking too fast, being emotionally charged, or not knowing what to say are stressors that cause us to stutter—to become tongue-tied—and this happens to us all. The stressor makes us "flustered" and we stutter. When we become "unflustered," that is, when the causes are addressed and removed, our speech returns to its normal cadence and flow.

Stuttering, the medical condition, is termed "developmental stuttering" to differentiate the condition from the occasional stuttering that affects us all. Developmental stuttering is not caused by speaking too fast, anger, confusion, nervousness, surprise, or being at loss for words, and does not resolve along with those situations. Speech patterns in developmental stuttering and being tongue-tied are similar, but the causes, course, and treatment are different. These differences define developmental stuttering and distinguish the condition from being tongue-tied.

Developmental Stuttering

Developmental stuttering, or stammering as the British refer to it, is an observed disruption in the normal fluency and mannerisms of speech. Fluent speech is considered to follow socially accepted time patterns, and stuttering is thus termed a "dysfluency" of speech in that there are breaks in the flow of speech. These dysfluencies of speech are the hallmark of developmental stuttering and distinguish the condition from other speech disorders.

Dysfluency has been recognized since ancient times. Egyptologists have deciphered two different hieroglyphics depicting stuttering and its dysfluency. The phonetic transcriptions of the hieroglyphics are ketket and nitit, meaning "to quake" and "to hesitate," respectively. When coupled with the Egyptian symbol indicating the mouth, the glyphs both translate "to stutter." The Egyptians were possibly the first to define stuttering speech, and did it by simple observation.

The current definition of developmental stuttering is similar to the first descriptions of the ancient Egyptians in that both are based on observations of the listener. However, unlike general descriptions of "quaking" or "hesitating" speech, modern medicine has discriminated specific speech patterns in those who stutter. Characteristic dysfluencies observed in developmental stuttering can be classified as occurring within words or between words or phrases.

Observation of those with developmental stuttering has revealed three dysfluencies that occur within words: sound and syllable repetitions, sound prolongations, and broken words:

sound and syllable repetitions
"Wh-Wh-What time is it?"

sound prolongations
"Wh———at time is it?"

broken words
"Wh (pause) at time is it?"

In addition to dysfluencies occurring within words, four characteristic dysfluencies disrupt the flow of speech between words: interjections, audible and silent blocking, circumlocutions, and monosyllabic whole-word repetitions:

interjections
"What ummmm time is it?"

audible and silent blocking (the person attempts to speak, while no or little sound is emitted)
"What (pause) time is it?"

circumlocutions (word substitutions to avoid problematic words or paraphrasing the intended sentence using different words)
"Wh—— Do you have the time?"

monosyllabic whole-word repetitions
"I-I-I have the time."

The above dysfluencies are the only ones observed in developmental stuttering. For example, multi-syllable repetitions do not occur. A mother admonishing a misbehaving child may become tongue-tied and shout "Jona-Jona-Jona-Jonathan!" The repetition of the two-syllable "Jona" is an example of stuttering speech but is not a characteristic of developmental stuttering.

When People Stutter

In addition to the specific types of dysfluencies found in developmental stuttering, the condition is defined by when these occur. Developmental stuttering is characterized by the occurrence of dysfluencies at the beginning of words and phrases. For example, a person with developmental stuttering would be much more prone to stutter the request, "Please pass the salt," as such:

P-P-P-Please pass the salt.

Whereas it would be quite unusual for the dysfluency to emerge in the latter part of the request:

Please pass the s-s-s-alt.

This aspect of stuttering helps differentiate developmental stuttering. Being tongue-tied does not have this specificity of occurrence. This specificity also contributes to one of the more frustrating manifestations of developmental stuttering: Stuttering occurs at the beginning of sentences. One of the more common times to stutter is when answering the phone; initiating the word "hello" can be difficult for those who stutter. This frustration is common for them, as it is reflective of a definitive symptom of the condition.

In developmental stuttering, the degree of stuttering can vary widely among individuals. Also, no matter if they stutter severely or just mildly, those who stutter tend to have "good days" and "bad days"—that is, a waxing and waning course of dysfluency.

Associated Symptoms

Dysfluencies are the core of developmental stuttering and are the bare minimum needed for diagnosis. Diagnosis is based on the type of dysfluency, when it occurs, and if it waxes and wanes over time. However, developmental stuttering is more than dysfluency. It is also associated with secondary motor behaviors and a form of anxiety termed "anticipatory anxiety." Most people who stutter have these symptoms to varying degrees, and the severest forms of developmental stuttering are most frequently accompanied by these associated symptoms, discussed below.

Secondary Motor Behaviors

In addition to the dysfluency, people who stutter may display secondary motor behaviors. A secondary motor behavior is an involuntary movement that occurs when one stutters. Motor tics, which are involuntary contractions of skeletal muscle, may accompany developmental stuttering. These tics commonly afflict the muscles of the face and neck. Rarely, contractions of muscles of the lower body may accompany developmental stuttering. Some who are afflicted with developmental stuttering may grind their feet into the ground or sway their whole body about.

Eye blinking, lip and tongue tremors, and disordered breathing are also common secondary motor behaviors. These behaviors are associated with developmental stuttering and are not separate medical conditions. If a person suffers from severe muscle contractions while stuttering, it may appear that he or she is having a seizure or is in respiratory distress. This is not the case. Muscle contractions are just one facet of the developmental stuttering phenomenon and their severity varies from person to person. The vignette below illustrates a typical presentation of a secondary motor behavior.

Bill was a fifteen-year-old boy who described his stuttering as severe and said he had been afflicted since he was five years old. He reported that in addition to his dysfluency, he would jerk his head to the side. This happened infrequently and only occurred when he was having a "bad stuttering day."

Bill came into my office because he had recently experienced a bad stuttering day at school. Bill stated that he was asked a question in class and stuttered when he answered. This stuttering was accompanied by a series of head jerks. As a result, Bill's classmates had made fun of him.

Bill wanted to know if there was a way he could predict when he would have a bad stuttering day. He did not want to go to school if he was going to have head jerks, and he said, "I'd rather take an F than get made fun of."

Secondary motor behaviors, head jerks in Bill's case, accompany severe dysfluency. As such, they wax and wane over time and there is no way to predict when they will emerge.

I explained to Bill that, unfortunately, there was no surefire way to tell when he would have a secondary motor behavior. I mentioned that if he was having a bad stuttering day, he should tell his teacher, so he would not be subjected to speaking in front of his classmates. I offered to write a letter to his teacher excusing him from class discussion during these times.

Bill accepted the offer and then asked if his head jerks were due to "nerves."

A common misconception is that associated secondary motor behaviors are due to "bottled up" anxiety. Anxiety is thought to be an evolutionary remnant of the "flight or fight" or "stress response." The stress response allows one to perform maximally during a threatening situation. When a person is confronted by a threat—for example, a pedestrian in a crosswalk whose path is soon to be crossed by an inattentive driver—the body prepares itself to best appraise and survive the danger. The pedestrian, when first noticing the oncoming car, immediately becomes more aware of and worried about the situation, breathes deeper, has an increase in heart rate and in energy, and sweats. These sensations are all due to the stress response, and in this example spur the pedestrian to move out of the car's way. The connection between the stress response and anxiety is that symptoms of stress resemble anxiety. Moreover, the brain areas that mediate the stress response are also implicated in anxiety. Involuntary muscle contractions serve no purpose in the stress response—a pedestrian does not need to have an involuntary leg kick or a head jerk while trying to escape a barreling car—and anxiety is not characterized by involuntary muscle contractions.

I told Bill that considering the circumstances at school and his calm, mature demeanor in my office, his "nerves" were in good shape. I reiterated that his head jerks are a symptom of his stuttering and not a separate manifestation caused by anxiety. However, I did explain that "nerves" can affect stuttering, and there is anxiety that is associated with developmental stuttering. He knew this and said,

"When I think about my stuttering, it makes it worse." I told him when he is thinking about his stuttering he is anticipating it. And this anticipation causes anxiety, which is termed "anticipatory anxiety."

Anticipatory Anxiety

Anticipatory anxiety is anxiety associated with the fear of stuttering. The fear of stuttering is directly proportional to the self-perception of communication. A person may stutter severely, but if he believes that he is communicating well and the audience is not distracted, he has less fear and hence less anticipatory anxiety. However, if he believes that his stuttering is affecting his ability to communicate, anticipatory anxiety emerges.

This anxiety can dominate a person's emotional life and is arguably the most socially inhibiting facet of developmental stuttering. Anticipatory anxiety is a result of stuttering and is cultivated by previous awkward social situations where one has felt embarrassed stuttering in the presence of others. This is a result of stuttering and not the cause. However, as anyone who has ever been scared knows, fear can impair one's ability to function, and anticipatory anxiety can exacerbate stuttering.

Anticipatory anxiety can significantly worsen the fluency and secondary motor behaviors of those who stutter. This anxiety does not cause developmental stuttering but is rather a catalyst for dysfluency. The memories of embarrassment and frustration of losing control of one's fluency are the seeds of anticipatory anxiety. When these memories are revisited, anxiety grows and as a result stuttering worsens. Anticipatory anxiety is a powerful force and will wring fluency away from the speaker brutally and without permission.

In summary, developmental stuttering is much more than being tongue-tied. Specific dysfluencies occur at the beginning of sentences or phrases. The degree of stuttering ranges widely from mild to severe. No matter the degree of stuttering, the person who stutters will have "good days" and "bad days." And, in addition to telltale dysfluencies, developmental stuttering is associated with secondary motor behaviors and anticipatory anxiety. This constellation of symptoms clearly distinguishes developmental stuttering from being tongue-tied and reveals that developmental stuttering is more than stuttering speech.

2. Who Stutters?

Developmental stuttering strikes children, typically emerging between the ages of two and six, and may continue throughout adulthood. Many successful and famous people have been afflicted with the condition. A short list includes writers Lewis Carroll and Somerset Maugham; moncarchs such as King George VI of England and King Louis II of France; scientists Robert Boyle and Erasmus Darwin; British mathematician Alan Turing, who created the theoretical model on which the modern computer is based and who deciphered the Nazi Enigma code during World War II; actress Marilyn Monroe; and contemporary figures such as country and western singer Mel Tillis, writer John Updike, athlete Bo Jackson, and actor James Earl Jones.

This list of accomplished people who stutter could continue for many pages and reflects their number in the general population. Listing the famous people who suffer from insulin-dependent diabetes would be just as impressive. (Whereas a list of the famous people who suffer from kuru, a dementia limited to three New Guinea tribes that is most likely spread by ritual cannibalism, would be quite sparse.) About one percent of the general population suffers from this type of diabetes; approximately the same percent of people stutter. Three million Americans are afflicted with developmental stuttering.

A Worldwide Phenomenon

Developmental stuttering is not confined to the western world. One percent of the world's population stutters and the condition affects every ethnicity and culture equally. This is best appreciated by the vast array of words that different cultures use to describe stuttering. In Ethiopia, the Amharic word is mentebateb. In Japan, domori is used. The Turks say kekelemek. All cultures recognize and have words that describe stuttering.

Interestingly, it has not been until recently that developmental stuttering was thought to be a cross-cultural, worldwide phenomenon. From 1937 to 1939, John C. Snidecor, head of the Department of Speech at the University of California, Santa Barbara, interviewed over eight hundred members of the Bannock-Shoshoni Indian tribe at the Fort Hall Reservation in Pocatello, Idaho. Snidecor also obtained data on more than one thousand other Bannock-Shoshoni, and "failed to find one pure-blooded Indian who stuttered."[1] Moreover, he reported that the tribal language had no word for stuttering. His conclusion was that the Bannock-Shoshoni did not stutter.

Snidecor's conclusion was published in the Quarterly Journal of Speech in 1947. This date is as significant as his findings, because in the 1940s there was a popular theory on the cause of developmental stuttering, and Snidecor's data—that the Bannock-Shoshoni did not stutter—supported this theory.

One proposed cause of developmental stuttering that was in vogue in the 1940s was the "diagnosogenic theory" of stuttering. Proponents of this theory believed that stuttering started when parents wrongly "diagnosed" their children with developmental stuttering. In this theory, the parents wronged not once, but twice. First, they would mistakenly diagnose as stuttering the normal dysfluencies children have as they learn language. They would follow this mistake with another by implementing remedies to control the stuttering. These remedies—it did not matter what they were—would be sensed by the child as disapproval. The child would then try to regain his parents' approval by speaking fluently. This would cause tension in the child, and the tension would cause the child to develop genuine stuttering.

There were two pieces of evidence from Snidecor's survey of the Bannock-Shoshoni that supported the diagnosogenic theory. One, since the Bannock-Shoshoni did not have a word for stuttering, they could not diagnose and admonish their children with the condition. Not having a word for stuttering would preclude the diagnosis and prevent the parents from giving their children the condition.

Two, the Bannock-Shoshoni "exert very little pressure upon the child to speak."[2] This lack of pressure was viewed as less tension on the child to speak fluently. Parents would not prematurely hasten the normal development of language and thus developmental stuttering would not develop.

The absence of stuttering in the Bannock-Shoshoni remained uncontested in the medical literature for some time. However, in 1983 an article from the Journal of Speech and Hearing Research set the record straight. Gerald Zimmerman, a professor of speech pathology at the University of Iowa, and his colleagues reported that the Bannock-Shoshoni had at least seventeen terms referring to stuttering. Examples include: kyc‡anni, meaning "to stutter;" pybyady, meaning "he stutters;" nicannugi/na, meaning "he stutters more and more," and so on. Snidecor never interviewed any Bannock-Shoshoni who stuttered because stuttering was stigmatized in the culture and the tribe never introduced to the doctor any people who stuttered. Zimmerman and his colleagues reported that the Bannock-Shoshoni "were embarrassed by members of their own families who stuttered."[3] Part of this embarrassment and stigmatization may be due to Bannock-Shoshoni folklore "attributing stuttering to the poorly executed passions of young couples."[4] Thus, like the western-derived diagnosogenic theory, the Bannock-Shoshoni also attributed stuttering to parents, albeit with a mitigating factor of passion.

The diagnosogenic theory eventually fell out of favor as it became known that developmental stuttering was not caused by admonishment to speak fluently. Now, officially including the Bannock-Shoshoni Indian tribe, it is known that about one percent of the world stutters—which means that 60 million people worldwide are afflicted with developmental stuttering.

Spontaneous Recovery

As stated earlier, the number of people with developmental stuttering is approximately the same as that of people who have insulin-dependent diabetes. But unlike diabetes, which in the majority of cases is a chronic, lifelong disease, many people who stutter do recover. This recovery means that developmental stuttering has afflicted more than one percent of the population.

In 1979, Kenneth Kidd and his colleagues from the Department of Human Genetics at the Yale University School of Medicine found that the approximate proportion of people in the general population who ever suffered from developmental stuttering is five percent. This means one out of twenty people have stuttered at some point during their life, whether they stutter now or not. This ratio does not include the normal dysfluencies of speech that everyone encounters from time to time. This five percent is a measure of bona fide developmental stuttering. This means that about fifteen million Americans are afflicted with the condition.

If five percent of the population has developmental stuttering at some time and one percent of the population currently stutters, then stuttering has an eighty percent spontaneous recovery rate. Spontaneous recovery is a rare event in medicine, and to have a condition that has an eighty percent spontaneous recovery rate is even rarer. This is definitely good news: the majority of children who stutter will recover completely before adulthood.

This high rate of spontaneous recovery is observed throughout the world. In addition, neither race nor culture has any affect on the spontaneous recovery rate. Eighty percent of those who stutter in Canada will recover, as well as those in China, in Cameroon, and so on.

However, age affects the spontaneous recovery rate. Developmental stuttering typically emerges between the ages of two and six, and most spontaneous recovery occurs during the elementary school years. Thus the older the children are, the more likely that they will not recover and will continue to stutter as adults.

In addition to age, spontaneous recovery is related to sex. When developmental stuttering is first diagnosed in children, more boys stutter than girls. The ratio is about two to one, and widens over time. By adulthood, the male-to-female ratio of the population who stutters is approximately four to one. Since developmental stuttering does not arise in adulthood, the widening of the ratio means that more girls recover from developmental stuttering than boys. Since fewer girls develop stuttering and those who do have a higher recovery rate, the end result is that most adults who stutter are male.

The Natural Course of Developmental Stuttering

The emergence of developmental stuttering is considered to be gradual. This onset occurs during the time period when children are learning language skills. Dysfluencies such as repeating syllables, hesitation, and syllable prolongation are a normal part of language development, and most children display symptoms of stuttering as they learn how to speak. Developmental stuttering is differentiated from the normal dysfluency encountered as a child learns language, when the dysfluency is accompanied by secondary motor behaviors such as facial tics, and by significant anxiety about speaking. Because dysfluencies are common in children, it takes time to distinguish between what is considered normal dysfluency and what is considered developmental stuttering. Over a period of time, it will become apparent whether or not a child truly has developmental stuttering.

In review, developmental stuttering is a cross-cultural, worldwide phenomenon that afflicts all types of people. One percent of the population stutters and five percent of the population has stuttered at some time. Thus in the United States, three million people currently stutter and fifteen million have stuttered at some time. Worldwide, the numbers are sixty million people and three hundred million people, respectively. For those afflicted, developmental stuttering begins gradually in childhood. Twice as many boys develop stuttering as girls, and girls have double the recovery rate. As a result, most adults who stutter are male.

The constellation of symptoms that is developmental stuttering afflicts a large group of people in a characteristic way. The onset of stuttering is gradual and the course is predictable. This is the nature of developmental stuttering. However, there is another condition called "acquired stuttering" that is of a completely different nature from that of developmental stuttering.

Acquired Stuttering

Developmental stuttering and acquired stuttering both include stuttering speech as a symptom, but they are dissimilar in many ways. Acquired stuttering is characterized by differences from developmental stuttering in prevalence, dysfluencies, onset, course, and recovery. The reason for these differences becomes apparent when the cause of acquired stuttering is explored.

Acquired stuttering is caused by an outside force—an environmental process—that affects brain function. Brain trauma, stroke, and even neurosurgical procedures can induce stuttering. Also, medications whose actions affect brain function can cause acquired stuttering. However, rarely do these events have stuttering as a symptom. For example, stroke affects about three-quarters of a million Americans each year and the numbers who have acquired stuttering as a result are few. In early 1990s, Arthur Grant and his colleagues from the Department of Neurology at the Emory University School of Medicine monitored how many stroke patients acquired stuttering at various hospitals affiliated with the medical school. Over a five-year period, treating thousands of patients, they reported only four cases. Acquired stuttering is rare, and even including all its various causes it is not nearly as common as developmental stuttering.

In addition to the difference in prevalence, the types of dysfluencies in acquired stuttering are different from those observed in developmental stuttering. In developmental stuttering, dysfluencies are confined to initial sounds and syllables alone. In acquired stuttering, dysfluencies are apparent throughout speech; even entire multisyllable words may be repeated. For example, a person who suffers from acquired stuttering may say "listening-ing-ing." This would never happen in a person who has developmental stuttering; a person with developmental stuttering may have difficulty saying a word but would never stutter on the last syllable. Moreover, acquired stuttering is not associated with secondary motor behaviors and anticipatory anxiety found in developmental stuttering.

Unlike developmental stuttering, the onset of acquired stuttering is usually acute, as with stroke, but there are cases of acquired stuttering emerging gradually. These cases are always associated with a slow-acting degenerative brain disease, such as Parkinson disease. As the disease progresses, the stuttering increases in frequency and intensity.

Because acquired stuttering is always associated with some type of brain insult, it usually presents in adults, who have had more time to injure themselves or develop disease. And most often, the oldest adults are afflicted with acquired stuttering, as they are the most susceptible to brain injury and have had the most time to develop an illness of the brain.

For example, in cases of stroke where there is permanent brain damage, the stuttering may be persistent. The prognosis for stuttering resolution is dependent on the severity of the process affecting brain function. In cases of severe brain disease, the prognosis is poor.

Acquired stuttering is quite different from developmental stuttering (Table 2.1). The only aspect that is similar is the stuttering, which is actually slightly different.

Table 2.1 Developmental vs. Acquired Stuttering		
	Developmental Stuttering	**Acquired Stuttering**
Types of dysfluency	specific	nonspecific
Occurence of dysfluency	at the beginning of speech	throughout speech
Onset	gradual	acute or gradual
Prevalence	common	very rare
Recovery	80%	varies

The Association between Developmental Stuttering and Tourette Syndrome

While acquired stuttering is not similar to developmental stuttering, Tourette syndrome is an illness that shares many characteristics with developmental stuttering. The similarities are striking, and make a comparison interesting and one wanting for explanation. Tourette syndrome was first described in 1885 by French neurologist George Gilles de la Tourette (1857–1904). The syndrome is defined by its two pathognomonic symptoms: motor and vocal tics. The tics in Tourette syndrome are involuntary, rapid, non-rhythmic muscle contractions and vocalizations. Motor tics in Tourette syndrome can affect any muscle group, but primarily involve muscles of the eye, head, and neck. Vocal tics are most commonly expressed as unintelligible sounds, which usually resemble a sniffing, grunting, or throat clearing sound. Less commonly vocal tics can be intelligible syllables or words. Rarely, albeit most famously, Tourette syndrome is associated with coprolalia, the utterance of obscenities.

Tourette syndrome affects four out of 10,000 children, the majority of which are boys. The numbers decline in adulthood to about 0.5 per 10,000. So, the course of Tourette syndrome is in parallel with developmental stuttering in that patients spontaneously recover, though the syndrome is 100 to 200 times less common than developmental stuttering.

In addition to following a similar course and having a predilection for males, the symptoms of Tourette syndrome share some other characteristics with developmental stuttering. In both conditions, symptoms wax and wane over time and vary in severity among afflicted individuals. Moreover, the tics in Tourette syndrome are involuntary and exacerbated by anxiety.

By sharing so many similarities, Tourette syndrome and developmental stuttering seem to be related. Possibly this relationship is that they share the same underlying mechanism, and Tourette syndrome may be just a variant of developmental stuttering. With this proposition, the question arises: Could they be the same condition?

This question has been addressed, and a genetic study has provided an answer. In 1993, David Pauls and his colleagues from the Child Study Center, Yale University School of Medicine examined the familial relationship between Tourette syndrome and developmental stuttering. Through extensive analysis of relatives of patients with both conditions, they concluded that Tourette syndrome and developmental stuttering are not the same genetic condition.

While the association between Tourette syndrome and developmental stuttering is strong, they are not the same. However, the understanding of both conditions has benefited from recent scientific advances, as both conditions are brain-based. Neuroscience research has shed some light on the cause of developmental stuttering and these discoveries are presented in the next chapter.

3. The Biology of Stuttering

Historical Views of Stuttering: The Role of the Tongue

Developmental stuttering is a genetic, brain-based condition. However, this understanding is only a recent phenomenon. Up until as late as the nineteenth century, a diseased tongue was considered the cause. For example, Biblical scholars believe that Moses stuttered and the book of Exodus (4:10) recounts how Moses was "slow of tongue." In the Midrashim, a collection of Talmudic stories, Moses' stutter is attributed to the burning of his tongue when he was a young boy. Ancient Greek and Roman physicians believed that developmental stuttering was caused by excessive moisture or dryness of the tongue. The famous Roman physician Galen (131–200 A.D.) recommended wrapping the tongue with cloth soaked in lettuce juice if a dry tongue caused the stuttering.

The Renaissance witnessed the revival of rational thinking and spurred progress in many aspects of medicine. Unfortunately for those who stuttered, the misconception of a diseased tongue as the root of developmental stuttering continued and all types of bizarre maneuvers were used as treatment for stuttering. Forks and wedges were placed below the tongue. Tubes were placed behind the tongue to eliminate the movements of the tongue during stuttering and to ensure proper airflow during speech. Neck belts were used to apply external pressure on the throat, which was thought to counteract the spasms of the tongue. Various exercises were promoted to increase the strength of the tongue and prevent spasms. Sadly, for a short time in the mid-nineteenth century, surgical excision of a wedge-shaped piece of the tongue was considered a successful treatment for stuttering.

Discovery of the Brain's Language Areas

By the twentieth century, the tongue was no longer thought to be the only culprit in stuttering. By this time, language production—as a process initiated by specific areas of the brain—was firmly imbedded in medical thought. Two discoveries clearly revealed that the brain controlled speech production. In 1862, French neurologist Pierre-Paul Broca (1801–1867) presented his autopsy findings of a 51-year-old patient who had lost the ability to speak around the age of 21. Broca demonstrated that the patient had a brain lesion in the left side of the brain. From this observation, Broca concluded that this area of the brain is necessary for the motor function of speech, in that it controls the motor movements of the speech apparatus that enable physical formation of words.

Later, in 1874, German psychiatrist Carl Wernicke (1848–1904) described another distinct area in the left side of the brain that when damaged caused disorganized speech. That is, patients with a lesion in this area were able to speak fluently, but the words did not follow conventional syntax and their speech had no meaning. These patients had lost the ability to associate the sounds they heard with the meanings of the words; therefore they had a sensory deficit of language. With these two discoveries—the motor area of speech (now termed Broca's area) and the sensory area of speech (now termed Wernicke's area)—the process of speech was localized to the left side of the brain.

These discoveries formed the template for the current understanding of developmental stuttering. Instead of investigation of end-stage organs of speech—such as the tongue—research is focused on describing stuttering as a dysfunction of areas in the brain involved in the process of speech. Within this framework, the brain mediates speech and thus mediates stuttering.

Basic Brain Structure and Function

The brain is divided into a number of specific anatomical regions. The largest and most highly developed area of the brain is the cerebrum. (Fig 3.1) The cerebrum regulates the most sophisticated mental functions, such as the senses, thinking, and movement, and is composed of two hemispheres. The left cerebral hemisphere contains the dominant areas for language, reasoning, and planning, and controls movement on the right side of the body. The right cerebral hemisphere is more specialized for musical abilities and the understanding of nonverbal symbols, and controls movement on the left side of the body. Directly below the cerebrum is the cerebellum; a bilateral structure involved with muscle tone and balance. In front of the cerebellum is the brain stem, which connects the spinal cord with the higher areas of the brain. The brain stem regulates the basic functions to sustain life, such as breathing and consciousness.

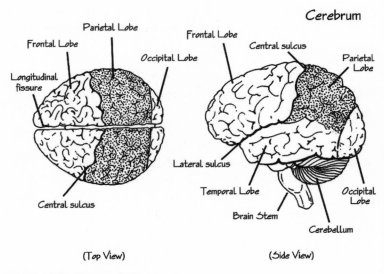

Fig 3.1 The Human Brain.

Each cerebral hemisphere is divided into four major portions termed lobes. The frontal lobes are involved with complex mental activities such as planning, reasoning, and immediate memory and also regulate voluntary motor movements. The frontal lobes are bounded by two clefts (sulci): the central sulcus at their posterior border and the lateral sulcus at their inferior border. The parietal lobes are involved with the processing of sensory information and are separated at their anterior border by the central sulcus and at their inferior border by the lateral sulcus. Adjacent to the posterior border of the parietal lobes are the occipital lobes, which interpret visual information. The temporal lobes are anterior to the occipital lobes and inferior to the frontal and parietal lobes. The temporal lobes are involved with memory, hearing, and emotions.

The outer area of each cerebral hemisphere and its collected lobes is called the cerebral cortex. The cerebral cortex has much surface area and, to fit within the confines of the skull, it folds upon itself. The resulting sulci demarcate the raised folds, termed "gyri." The cerebral cortex has connections, direct or indirect, with all parts of the body.

Enclosed by each cerebral hemisphere are the deep structures of the brain. (Fig 3.2) These include the basal ganglia, the amygdala, and the thalamus. The components of the basal ganglia are the caudate, globus pallidus, and the putamen. These structures are involved in the regulation of motor movements. Connected to the tail of the caudate is the amygdala. The amygdala is involved in anxiety, aggression, and the formation of memory. Adjacent to the basal ganglia is the thalamus, which processes and filters sensory information.

Other important areas deep within the brain are the cingulate gyrus, found on the inner part of each hemisphere and involved with emotions and motivated behavior; the corpus callosum, a band of neurons that connects the cerebral hemispheres; the hypothalamus, which regulates body temperature, hunger, and the release of hormones from glands; the hippocampus, located in the inferior portion of each cerebral hemisphere and concerned with memory; the fornix, a tract of nerve fibers that connects the hippocampus

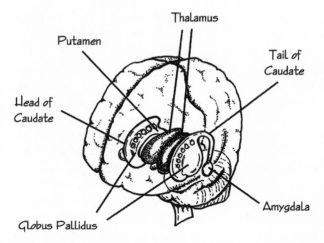

Fig 3.2 Deep Brain Structures: Amygdala, Basal Ganglia, and Thalamus. The Lobes of the Cerebral Hemispheres.

with the hypothalamus; and the pituitary gland, which is located at the base of the cerebral hemispheres and releases hormones that regulate a number of biochemical processes, such as growth and metabolism.

Communication within the various areas of the brain is mediated by neurons, which are the cells that make up the brain. A neuron consists of a cell body surrounded by dendrites. Dendrites allow the neuron to receive information from other neurons. This information is propagated along the neuron through the axon via electrical impulses. The axon branches out as it terminates, and these axon terminals may connect with dendrites of other neurons.

Communication among neurons is via "neurotransmitters." Neurotransmitters are molecules that transfer neuronal impulses from cell to cell, and this communication occurs at the space where the axon terminal of one neuron connects with the dendrite of another. This space is termed the "synapse." When a neuron passes its electrical message along the axon, neurotransmitters are released from storage vesicles in the axon terminals. Once released into the synapse, neurotransmitters diffuse across and attach to receptors.

Depending on the type of neurotransmitter and the type of receptor it binds to, the recipient brain cells will be more or less apt to discharge an electrical message.

There are many different types of neurotransmitters and each neurotransmitter is associated with receptors that have different functions. Examples of well-studied neurotransmitters are acetylcholine, dopamine, norepinephrine, and serotonin.

Language Areas of the Brain

Language is the ability to speech, listen, read, and write, and in ninety-nine percent of individuals is located in the left cerebral hemisphere. The dominance of language is more pronounced than the dominance of handedness. Ninety percent of individuals are right-handed and have more skill and dexterity initiating and performing motor movements with the right side of their body. All of these individuals are left cerebral hemisphere dominant for language and handedness. In addition, most individuals who are left-handed—who are right cerebral dominant for handedness—have a dominant left cerebral hemisphere for language. The association of handedness and developmental stuttering is the same as that found in the general population—that is, the vast majority of those who stutter are right-handed.

The brain processes language in a systematic fashion. The ears transform sound waves to neuronal impulses and these impulses are transmitted to the primary auditory cortex in each temporal lobe (Fig 3.3). Language impulses from both primary auditory cortices are then delivered to Wernicke's area, which is located in the superior gyrus of the left temporal lobe. Wernicke's area associates these impulses with words to give the impulses a meaning. Once this association occurs, the impulses travel along the arcuate fasciculus—an arc of nerve fibers that pass through the temporal, parietal, and frontal lobes—to Broca's area, which is located in the frontal lobe. Broca's area receives these integrated language impulses and is able to articulate these impulses by activating areas of the brain that

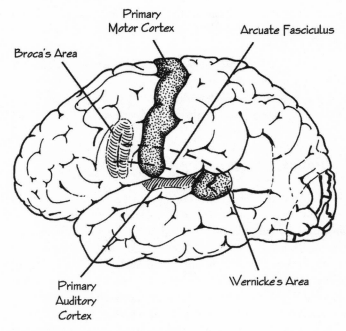

Fig 3.3 The Languages Areas of the Brain.

control speech (such as the larynx, lips, and tongue), which are located in the primary motor cortex of the frontal lobe.

For example, when one is asked to repeat the word "book," the sound of the word "book" is first heard by the ears and transformed into nerve impulses. At this point in the language system these impulses have no meaning, so the person cannot yet identify that the sound impulses represent the word "book." However, once these impulses are transmitted to Wernicke's area they are recognized as having a meaning, and the person understands that they have been asked to repeat a specific word.

In order to complete the task, the nerve impulses—that are now associated with "book"—travel to Broca's area. Broca's area understands this nerve transmission as a specific word and dictates the motor areas of the brain to say "book."

All language activity is processed by these areas of the brain, and recent research suggests that developmental stuttering is associated with variations in the brain areas associated with language.

Stuttering and the Brain: Neuroimaging

Recent scientific discoveries have provided significant understanding of the brain processes that mediate developmental stuttering. One of the most amazing scientific breakthroughs in developmental stuttering is the recent ability to study the living human brain. Neuroimaging techniques allow this study and these techniques are categorized as "functional" or "structural." Functional neuroimaging techniques permit examination of brain activity as a function of time, which provides information on how physical and mental processes are organized and performed by the brain. Structural neuroimaging techniques permit examination of the detailed structure of the living brain. These techniques are one of the most powerful tools in psychiatric research, and have provided a wealth of new information concerning brain function and developmental stuttering.

Functional Neuroimaging Techniques

Four different functional neuroimaging techniques have been applied to developmental stuttering: electroencephalography (EEG), magnetoencephalography (MEG), single-photon emission computed tomography (SPECT), and positron emission tomography (PET). Each of these functional neuroimaging techniques has its own advantages, which are primarily related to the resolution of brain activity obtained with each technique.

As a brief introduction, EEG and MEG are functional neuroimaging techniques that directly measure electrical communication between neurons. These two techniques provide excellent temporal resolution; they can detect changes in brain activity over very short periods of time. However, they have poor spatial resolution, meaning they have less ability to discern which areas of the brain are activated. SPECT and PET are techniques that use "tracers" to measure blood and chemical activity in the brain. The tracers used in SPECT and PET emit a detectable signal, and this signal is used to determine brain activity. SPECT is an older technology than PET and has less resolution. For research purposes, PET has replaced SPECT. PET does not have the temporal resolution of EEG or MEG, but has better spatial resolution.

All of the above-mentioned functional neuroimaging techniques have been or are being used to observe brain function in developmental stuttering. They have provided evidence of functional differences in the brains of those who stutter.

EEG Studies of Developmental Stuttering

EEG measures the direct electrical activity of neurons via electrodes placed on the scalp. The benefit of EEG is that these electrodes can detect changes in brain activity by the millisecond, and thus provides excellent temporal resolution. However, because the electrodes are on the scalp, the detection of the electrical activity is less sensitive for deep areas of the brain, and even with current technology EEG has the poorest spatial resolution of all the function neuroimaging techniques, with a spatial resolution of 10 to 15 millimeters.

EEG was the first functional neuroimaging technique developed, and was the first neuroimaging technique to reveal that brain activity is different in those who stutter. In 1967, Drs. S. Schmoigl and W. Ladisich of Innsbruck, Austria, obtained EEGs from 50 individuals with developmental stuttering at rest and observed diffuse generalized changes in 70 percent of the EEGs. The results did not localize an area of the brain associated with developmental stuttering—as the methodology and EEG technology at the time did not lend themselves to such a discovery—but they offered their findings as evidence that developmental stuttering has a neurological component. This study provided the first view of the living brain and suggested that developmental stuttering is related to differences in brain activity.

In 1974, Gerald Zimmermann and J. R. Knott from the Department of Psychiatry at the University of Iowa presented the first EEG study assessing brain activity in developmental stuttering while individuals spoke. They examined nine individuals with developmental stuttering and compared the results with a control group of fluent speakers. All of these individuals were right-handed, and therefore left cerebral dominant for language. In 78 percent of patients in the developmental stuttering group, they found more electrical activity in the right cerebral hemisphere than the left when speaking. This contrasted with their observation that only 20 percent of fluent speakers demonstrated this type of pattern. With this work, Zimmerman and Knott concluded that there are hemispheric differences in brain activity in those who stutter, and were the first to use neuroimaging to localize differences in brain activity in those who stutter.

EEG studies in the 1970s and 1980s confirmed there were hemispheric differences in brain activity in those who stutter. The general conclusions were that those with developmental stuttering have greater right hemisphere brain activity, or a decrease in left hemisphere activity, when processing language compared to fluent speakers. This is a significant finding, as the language areas of the brain are located in the left hemisphere and those who stutter do not employ the language areas of the brain with the same robust activity as those who are fluent. However, the limitations in spatial resolution of this period of EEG research did not lend to a consensus on the specific locations of where these changes occurred within the cerebral hemispheres.

Modern EEG is still hindered by limited spatial resolution. Over the past decade, EEG has been replaced by more sophisticated neuroimaging techniques that provide more detailed spatial resolution, and thus can localize brain activity with more precision. One of these techniques is MEG.

MEG Studies of Developmental Stuttering

MEG measures neuronal activity by the millisecond through detection of magnetic fields produced by neuronal electrical current. Sensors placed on the scalp detect these magnetic fields, and as with EEG, brain activity closest to the scalp is more easily localized. The measurement of magnetic fields does provide a benefit in that spatial resolution is about 5 millimeters.

However, a factor that limits MEG use is that the machines are very expensive, in part because the sensors have to be kept very cold and protected from outside magnetic fields. In order to detect the small magnetic fields arising from active neurons, the sensors are enclosed in a helmet that is filled with liquid helium, which keeps the sensors at a superconducting temperature of -269 degrees Celsius. In addition, MEG is performed in shielded rooms that prevent interfering magnetic fields. Unfortunately, these limitations prevent many researchers from using MEG. Nonetheless, MEG has been used in developmental stuttering, and the two MEG studies of developmental stuttering have provided the most detailed information to date on the millisecond-by-millisecond changes in brain activity that occur in the condition.

Riitta Salmelin and her colleagues from the Brain Research Unit at the Helsinki University of Technology have used MEG to study how the brain processes language in those who stutter. In 1998, Salmelin and her colleagues compared the response of the auditory cortex (Fig 3.3) to auditory stimuli in nine individuals with developmental stuttering and a control group performing multiple tasks: while they were reading silently, with mouth movements only, aloud, and in chorus with another person. The auditory stimuli were used to prompt activity within the language areas of the brain, and the different tasks were employed to highlight specific areas within the language circuit. For example, when reading silently there is no increase in neuronal activity in Broca's area because the words are not articulated. During this study, they found no difference in timing of brain activity between the developmental stuttering group and the control group, in that both groups had the same brain activity about 100 milliseconds after stimulation. However, they found that auditory stimulation of the right and left auditory cortices during the tasks provoked variable patterns of activity between the right and left auditory cortices when compared to the control group. From this observation, they offered that the means by which the auditory cortex processes language might be different in those who stutter.

In 2000, Salmelin and her colleagues expanded on these findings by using a different technique to explore the cerebral activation patterns in developmental stuttering. They compared groups of the same size as in their previous study while the participants read single words. This methodology allowed a comparison of fluent speech production between the two groups, as the group with developmental stuttering was able to read the single words fluently. Interestingly, even with the end result being fluent speech, the cortical activation patterns were clearly different between the groups. Within the first 0.4 seconds after seeing the word, brain activity was observed in the left hemisphere in both groups, but the sequence was opposite. In the control group, the brain activity was found to flow from Broca's area to the dorsal premotor cortex (which can assist in the motor execution of articulation and is located in the frontal lobe anterior to the primary motor cortex) and the primary motor cortex. This is a normal pattern of activation of the language circuit. However, in the developmental stuttering group the sequence of brain activation was reversed at the last stages of the language circuit. When speaking, the dorsal premotor cortex and the primary motor cortex showed activity before Broca's area was activated. Those with developmental stuttering appeared to initiate motor movements of words before receiving how to articulate the words from Broca's area. In addition, they reported the same generalized pattern of activity found in the previous EEG studies in that speech production elicited more brain activity in the nondominant right cerebral hemisphere.

These MEG studies showed that brain activity in developmental stuttering responds as fast as in those without, but in a different manner. Those who stutter appear to have a different means by which to process language in the auditory cortices and activate language areas in the brain in a different order from those who do not stutter. These differences in brain activity were not detected by earlier EEG studies, a reflection of the superior temporal resolution of MEG compared to EEG and the skill of the researchers. However, the limitations of MEG are its spatial resolution—especially for structures deep within the brain. SPECT and PET can provide better spatial resolution, and these modalities have provided more information on how the brain functions in developmental stuttering.

SPECT Studies of Developmental Stuttering

SPECT uses radioactive tracers that emit single photons to form an image. These tracers are commonly used to measure blood flow in the brain. This is a secondary means by which to measure brain activity, as increased cerebral blood flow is a sign of increased neuronal activity. The temporal resolution of SPECT is about one minute and the spatial resolution is from 6 to 8 millimeters, which is less resolution than the newer technology of PET. Although PET has replaced SPECT as a research tool, the first two functional neuroimaging studies measuring blood flow in developmental stuttering were by SPECT. The results from these two SPECT studies provided a foundation for future neuroimaging queries.

In 1980, Frank Wood and his colleagues at Wake Forest University Medical Center reported the first SPECT study in developmental stuttering. The study consisted of two adults who stuttered who underwent SPECT scans before and after taking haloperidol. Haloperidol is a medication that induces fluency. (Haloperidol is discussed in detail in Chapter 4.) Before treatment with haloperidol, Wood and his colleagues observed increased blood flow to the right cerebral hemisphere when the individuals spoke. This observation was consistent with prior EEG work. Interestingly, after haloperidol administration, blood flow reversed and more activity was detected in the left cerebral hemisphere. They interpreted these results as evidence that developmental stuttering is

associated with inadequate left cerebral dominance for speech production, and that haloperidol corrected this.

In 1991, Kenneth Pool and his colleagues at the University of
Texas Southwestern Medical Center reported their results using
SPECT to assess cerebral blood flow in 20 adults with developmental stuttering while silent. They compared the SPECT results to a
control group and found that the group with developmental stuttering had more blood flow to three areas in the right hemisphere and
less blood flow throughout the brain when compared to controls.
They offered these results as preliminary evidence that developmental stuttering is related to reduced and asymmetric perfusion of
the brain.

PET Studies of Developmental Stuttering

By the mid-1990s, PET had replaced SPECT as the predomi-
nant functional neuroimaging tool, as PET offers more precision
than SPECT. Like SPECT, PET relies on the use of tracers to form
images. These tracers emit positrons, which are similar to electrons
in that they are subatomic particles, but are positively charged. The
tracers provide a benefit in that they can be attached to other molecules, such as glucose and neurotransmitters, to study specific brain
processes as well as the indirect brain activity via blood flow. PET
offers good temporal resolution—about 45 seconds—and the spatial resolution is approximately 4 millimeters. And unlike EEG or
MEG, PET can measure the activity of deep brain structures.

The disadvantage of using PET, as with SPECT, is that these
tracers are radioactive. The danger associated with this radioactivity
is small, but there are safety regulations that limit how many times a
person can be exposed to the radiation. Also, PET machines are
very expensive, so obtaining scans is costly. The cost of PET limits
the number of patients who can be scanned in a study and the total
amount of studies undertaken.

As of this writing, eight PET studies have addressed brain function in developmental stuttering—a relatively small number

compared with the fifty-eight EEG studies that have been performed. These PET studies have been performed by four different groups: Joseph Wu and his colleagues from the Department of Psychiatry at the University of California, Irvine; the collaboration of Peter Fox and his colleagues from the Research Imaging Center at the University of Texas Health Science Center with Roger Ingham his colleagues from the Department of Speech and Hearing Sciences at the University of California, Santa Barbara; Allen Braun and his colleagues from the National Institute on Deafness and Other Communication Disorders, National Institutes of Health; and Luc DeNil and his colleagues from the Department of Speech-Language Pathology at the University of Toronto. As expected when comparing a small number of research studies that employ different designs and a small number of patients, there are conflicting results. Each study has viewed stuttering from different vantage points, and accordingly has observed a different perspective. However, no matter the vantage point, there is an observation that is uniform among these different PET studies: that brain function in developmental stuttering is associated with differences in hemispheric asymmetry in the cerebral cortex, and specifically that the right cerebral cortex is more active in those who stutter. This is the same finding noted in EEG and MEG studies. In addition, observations of the deep brain structures (Fig 3.2), namely the caudate, the cerebellum, and cingulate gyrus, reveal that deep brain structures show different activity in individuals with developmental stuttering compared to fluent speakers.

Structural Neuroimaging

For hundreds of years, investigation of the brain's anatomical structure in patients with developmental stuttering revealed no difference between those and the brains of fluent speakers. This lack of difference has historical significance as it prompted misguided views concerning the role of the tongue in stuttering and gave credence to a variety of psychological explanations for stuttering, like the diagnosogenic theory presented in Chapter 2. With the emergence of magnetic resonance imaging (MRI), the most powerful structural neuroimaging technique available, a centuries-old assumption has been reevaluated. MRI has revealed some slight differences in brain structure in those who stutter.

MRI is based on the principle of nuclear magnetic resonance, which was first described in 1946 by the American physicists Felix Block (1905–1983) and Edward Purcell (1912–1997). (In 1952 they were awarded a Nobel Prize for their discovery.) Nuclear magnetic resonance describes the behavior of protons in a magnetic field. A proton is a positively charged unit that resides in the nucleus of all atoms. The simplest atom is the hydrogen atom, which consists of only one proton. Since water comprises more than half of the human body and water is composed of two atoms of hydrogen and one atom of oxygen (H^2O), there are many hydrogen atoms in the human body. Moreover, the molecules that constitute most of the non-water components of the human body—proteins, carbohydrates, and fat—contain many hydrogen atoms. The abundance of hydrogen atoms in the human body is fortunate, as MRI is possible due to the nuclear magnetic resonance of a hydrogen atom.

When a person undergoes MRI, he or she is placed in a scanner that produces a very strong magnetic field. (Most MRI machines have magnets that generate a magnetic field of 1.5 Tesla, which is about 150 times as strong as the average refrigerator magnet.) Being in this strong magnetic field causes the hydrogen atoms in the body to align in accordance with the magnetic field. This magnetic alignment is the baseline state of the MRI procedure. After magnetization occurs, radio waves are directed at the person, which is a safe procedure as radio waves are harmless; we are bombarded with them every day by radio stations without ill effect. Magnetized hydrogen atoms will resonate at the frequency of radio waves, hence the term magnetic resonance. This period of hydrogen atom resonance is the excitation or activation state of MRI. After excitation, the radio waves are stopped and the hydrogen atoms return to their baseline state. The key step for image formation is that when the hydrogen atoms return to baseline they emit radio waves.

Depending on the local environment the hydrogen atom is in, that is, the type of tissue, the rate of radio wave emission is different. These different radio wave frequencies are then detected by the MRI scanner and reconstructed to form an image on a computer screen. These images then can be printed out on film and are the most detailed view of the living brain available to modern medicine.

In 2001, Anne Foundas and her colleagues from the Departments of Psychiatry and Neurology at Tulane University obtained brain MR images from 16 adults with developmental stuttering and MR images from a control group. When they compared the volumes of the individuals who stutter versus those who did not, they found that many of these patients had slight differences in brain anatomy. Foundas and her colleagues observed enlarged planum temporale, which is a cortical area of the brain that includes Wernicke's area, in the group with developmental stuttering. Enlarged planum temporale were found in both cerebral hemispheres and thus there was less asymmetry between the dominant and nondominant hemispheres. Asymmetry of the planum temporale is considered a normal MRI finding in persons without language problems, as this area is associated with language and typically has greater cortical area than its nondominant conterpart (Fig 3.4). In addition, the researchers observed differences in gyral patterns throughout the cortical speech language areas between the two groups. (Gyral patterns are a common way to note brain anatomy.) Foundas and her colleagues found that the gyral pattern differences in the developmental stuttering group were more apparent in the frontal regions of the brain, which includes Broca's area. In analysis of these anatomical differences, there was not one specific anatomical difference in size or gyral pattern particular to the individuals who stuttered. However, based on these overall differences in brain structure, Foundas and her colleagues could differentiate between the group with developmental stuttering and the control group.

The results of this study provide the first evidence that adults with developmental stuttering have anatomical variations in brain

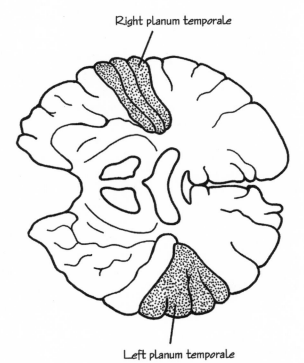

Axial view of Brain with Frontal Lobes removed revealing
normal asymmetry of Planum Temporale

Fig 3.4 Planum Temporale.

areas associated with speech. The variations are slight and no one
anatomical variation is particular to those who stutter, but this
study outlines a structural map of brain areas that mediate developmental stuttering that corresponds with the observations noted in
the functional neuroimaging studies.

Brain areas involved with formulation and expression of language, which in the vast majority of individuals are located in the
dominant left cerebral hemisphere, appear to be expressed in the
right hemisphere or bilaterally in those who stutter. This finding is

not exclusive to developmental stuttering. Other conditions that involve disruptions of language or communication, such as dyslexia, autism, delayed speech, and Asperger's syndrome are noted to have more right cerebral hemisphere involvement and a lack of planum temporale asymmetry.

In addition to increased area and activity of the right cerebral hemisphere, those who stutter appear to activate language areas in the left cerebral hemisphere in a different order from those who do not stutter. Specifically, those with developmental stuttering may begin speaking before the brain dictates how the words should be articulated.

By peering into the living brain, neuroimaging has shown that the brain is undoubtedly involved in developmental stuttering. Specific patterns of activation and areas have been implicated via these studies. As the technology improves, as is happening right now, a clearer picture of brain function will emerge, and the future for further breakthroughs is bright.

Observations of Acquired Stuttering: Pharmacology and Disease

Another facet of science that has contributed to the medical conceptualization of developmental stuttering is observations of acquired stuttering. Along with neuroimaging, the understanding of brain function in developmental stuttering has been furthered by observations of acquired stuttering. To review, acquired stuttering is caused by outside forces that affect brain function. Interestingly, there are certain pharmacological compounds and diseases that can induce acquired stuttering, and even diminish stuttering speech. By studying the actions of these forces, the neural mechanisms that mediate the stuttering state can be deduced. This is of help in understanding the underlying cause of developmental stuttering, as it adds insight into the inner workings of stuttering speech.

Psychopharmacology and the Role of Dopamine

Psychopharmacology refers to the effects of medication on brain function. The induction of stuttering by medicines known to affect brain function, and the subsequent return of fluency when these medications are discontinued, is evidence that the part of the brain affected may be involved in stuttering speech. A wide variety of medications with many different mechanisms of action have been reported to induce stuttering speech as a rare side effect, but only a few medications—that share a similar mechanism of action—commonly induce stuttering speech. Science relies on reproducible results, so the scientific focus has been directed toward the small group of medications that consistently induce stuttering speech. This focus has revealed that these medications increase dopaminergic activity in the brain.

Amphetamines and levodopa are medications that can cause acquired stuttering as a side effect, and both increase dopamine in the brain. Amphetamines increase dopaminergic activity in the brain primarily by facilitating the release of dopamine from storage vesicles in the axon terminal into the synapse. This action causes an increase of dopamine in the synaptic cleft, which increases electrical transmission between the neurons. Amphetamines are commonly used in treating attention-deficit/hyperactivity disorder, in that increased dopaminergic activity in the brain increases the ability to focus. Levodopa is a precursor of dopamine and increases dopaminergic activity by increasing the amount of dopamine synthesized in the neuron. Levodopa is used to restore the depleted dopamine in patients with Parkinson disease, which is associated with a deterioration of dopaminergic neurons in the brain.

The association of these medications and stuttering helps with the understanding of how the brain mediates stuttering as dopaminergic neurons are localized in specific areas of the brain. The dopamine system in the brain is divided into four discrete pathways (Fig. 3.5). One pathway arises in the hypothalamus and projects to the pituitary gland. This pathway is involved in the

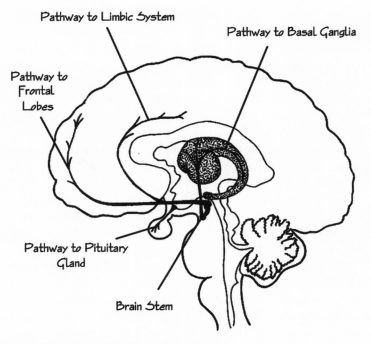

Fig 3.5 Dopaminergic Pathways in the Brain.

regulation of the hormone prolactin. Prolactin helps mediate lactation and ovulation. The other three pathways arise from the brain stem. One pathway projects to the limbic system. The limbic system is an evolutionally old area deep within the brain that is associated with emotions and drives. Dopaminergic neurons from this pathway have been implicated in addiction. Another pathway projects primarily to frontal lobes of the cortex, and plays a role in schizophrenia. The last pathway projects to the basal ganglia. The basal ganglia help regulate motor movements, and deterioration of this dopaminergic pathway causes the tremors and shuffling gait observed in Parkinson disease.

Amphetamines and levodopa enter the brain and increase dopaminergic activity throughout the dopamine system. When stuttering arises as a side effect of these medications, increased dopamine is the likely cause. Since the dopaminergic system is limited to certain areas of the brain, the brain mechanism for stuttering speech in these cases is confined to the four pathways. Which pathways contribute to stuttering speech is unknown; however, the pathway that projects to the frontal lobe, which houses Broca's area and other areas associated with speech, and the pathway that projects to the basal ganglia, which regulates motor movements and is implicated via PET studies in developmental stuttering, appear to be to the most likely ones involved in stuttering speech.

Disease and the Role of the Thalamus

Head trauma and stroke have been associated with new onset stuttering. Observations of where the damage in the brain has occurred have not revealed a specific area where damage induces stuttering speech. For example, there are multiple reports of patients with strokes who develop stuttering speech, having lesions affecting different areas of the brain. Reviews of case reports of stuttering speech and brain injury have not been very helpful in identifying areas of the brain specific to stuttering speech. However, an incidental finding during a neurosurgical procedure revealed that the thalamus plays a role in stuttering speech.

The thalamus is an area deep within the center of the brain that has connections with almost every other part of the brain (Fig 3.2). The thalamus is a small region, with a volume of about 12 cubic centimeters. The primary role of the thalamus is to process sensory information throughout the brain. Simply put, the thalamus filters all the sensations to the brain and mediates which information should be suppressed or communicated to other areas of the brain.

Being that the thalamus is in the center of the brain, its activity is not well detected with functional neuroimaging techniques that use sensors on the scalp, such as EEG and MEG. Moreover, since the thalamus functions as a sensory filter, it is difficult to devise experimental paradigms that are directed at monitoring its activity. Thus, activity of the thalamus in developmental stuttering has not been consistently observed in SPECT or PET neuroimaging studies.

In 1989, Subhash Bhatnagar and Orlando Andy from the Department of Speech Pathology and Audiology at Marquette University and the Department of Neurosurgery at the University of Mississippi Medical Center, respectively, reported of an individual with intractable pain arising from the trigeminal nerve, which is a nerve that innervates the face. This patient's pain had become progressively worse over a 20-year period, and previous medication regimens and surgical techniques had failed to alleviate the pain. Other than the severe chronic pain, the patient developed stuttering speech over the years. As a treatment of last resort, the patient underwent a neurosurgical procedure where an electrode was implanted in the thalamus to disrupt the transmission of the pain. This surgery was a success, and the patient's pain subsided. As a side effect of the surgery, the patient's speech became fluent and this fluency continued as the patient's thalamus was stimulated by the electrode.

Two years later, Bhatnagar and Andy reported of another patient who underwent thalamic surgery for chronic pain. As in the previous patient, the surgery successfully relieved the pain. However, in the course of the procedure, the patient developed stuttering speech when the same region of the thalamus was surgically destroyed. In the course of two years, Bhatnagar and Andy had reported the alleviation of stuttering speech with stimulation of the thalamus and the emergence of stuttering when the same area of the thalamus was destroyed.

These observations implicate the thalamus in the production of stuttering speech. Since the thalamus only processes sensory information, it cannot initiate the motor aspects of stuttering. However, as the thalamus has connections throughout the brain, it possibly is involved in the stuttering phenomenon through its connections with the motor speech producing areas.

Genetics

Familial Studies of Developmental Stuttering

Familial studies reveal that developmental stuttering runs in families: those with developmental stuttering have a much higher incidence of having a family history of stuttering than does the general population. From the 1920s to 1983 there were 23 familial studies of developmental stuttering. In these studies, the average percentage for a family history of stuttering in those who stutter ranges from 30 percent to 60 percent, whereas the average percentage of family history of stuttering in those who do not stutter is less than 10 percent. The wide range of percentages found in summarizing the medical literature of past familial studies reflects the wide range of study designs used by the different researchers. For example, over the years researchers have used different criteria to diagnose developmental stuttering, and this contributes to fluctuations in percentages.

More recent familial studies, which have used contemporary definitions of developmental stuttering, have given more specific results. In 1991, Marie Poulos and William Webster from the Ottawa Rehabilitation Centre, Ontario, thoroughly screened 169 adolescents and adults who stuttered for any evidence of acquired stuttering and separated them from those with developmental stuttering. From this group, 145 met strict criteria for a diagnosis of developmental stuttering. Of those with developmental stuttering, 75.2 percent had a family history of stuttering, whereas only 14.3 percent of the individuals with suspected acquired stuttering had a family history significant for stuttering.

In 1993, Nicoline Ambrose and her colleagues from the University of Illinois at Urbana-Champaign also incorporated strict diagnostic criteria in analyzing the family history of those with developmental stuttering. In this study, Ambrose and her colleagues investigated 69 children with developmental stuttering. They obtained detailed family trees from the parents of these children. Since most of the relatives of these children were living, they were able to ask family members if they ever stuttered. This allowed confirmation of a diagnosis of developmental stuttering in these relatives. Ambrose and her colleagues found that a child who stutters has a 42 percent chance of having an immediate family member with developmental stuttering. Moreover, if the family tree is expanded to include second and third degree relatives, the child who stutters has a 71 percent chance of having an extended family member with developmental stuttering.

Familial studies of developmental stuttering, while varying to some degree, show a high association between the expression of developmental stuttering and having a family history of the condition. This strong association lends evidence to a genetic component to developmental stuttering. However, just because developmental stuttering appears more frequently in the families of those who stutter than would be expected in the general population does not prove that developmental stuttering is genetic.

All genetic illnesses show a familial history; however, so can other illness that do not have a genetic component. Environmentally caused illness such as infections and nutritional deficiencies can appear to have a genetic distribution, in that these conditions can be clustered in families. Thus, familial studies only suggest a genetic component. Interestingly, the first familial studies of developmental stuttering were used to support an environmentally attributed cause. The diagnosogenic theory of stuttering required the parental transmission of verbal admonishment, and its supporters found comfort in observing the high familial incidence in those who stuttered.

Even though familial studies do not prove a genetic basis to diseases and traits, they do support the postulation and give credence to further genetic inquiry. One way to distinguish genetic causes from environmental causes is to study identical twins.

Twin Studies of Developmental Stuttering

The power of twin studies relies on that fact that identical (monozygotic) twins share 100 percent of their genes. Fraternal (dizygotic) twins share 50 percent of their genes. This difference in genetic constitution between twin types is helpful in genetic studies of twins, because if there is a genetic component to an illness or trait it should be expressed significantly more in monozygotic twins than in dizygotic twins. Twin studies of developmental stuttering have revealed that this is the case.

In 1981, Pauline Howie from the University of New South Wales, Sydney, analyzed all of the published twin studies of developmental stuttering. She found eleven studies, with the first study performed in 1945. Analysis of the results from all of these studies revealed that 78 percent of identical twins were "concordant" for stuttering. Concordant means that if one twin stutters, the other twin also stutters. Analysis revealed that fraternal twins were only 9 percent concordant for stuttering.

Howie also performed her own study. She studied 30 twin pairs of which 17 were identical and 13 were fraternal. She found that 63 percent of the identical twins were concordant for stuttering, whereas only 19 percent of the fraternal twins were concordant.

The most recent twin study in the medical literature also supports this pattern. Susan Felsenfeld from the Department of Speech-Language Pathology, Duquesne University, Pittsburgh, and her colleagues from the Virginia Institute for Psychiatric and Behavior Genetics, Richmond, and the Queensland Institute of Medical Research, Queensland, Australia, examined twin pairs from the Australian Twin Registry. Felsenfeld and her colleagues interviewed 38 identical twins and 53 fraternal twins where at least one twin had developmental stuttering. They found 45 percent concordance for developmental stuttering in the identical twins and only 15 percent concordance in the fraternal twins.

All of the twin studies of developmental stuttering show an increased concordance for the condition in identical twins when compared with fraternal twins. However, a proven genetic background does not necessarily mean that other factors are not relevant to developmental stuttering. If it did, concordance in identical twins would be 100 percent. Thus, a multitude of environmental factors must influence the emergence of developmental stuttering in those genetically predisposed to it.

4. Treatments for Stuttering

There is no easy way, with present diagnostic techniques, to diagnose developmental stuttering in young children. Consequently, it is difficult to determine when it is appropriate to refer children for treatment. On one hand, one wants to make sure all children who need treatment receive it, and on the other hand, one does not want to cause unneeded worry and expense to families. Achieving this balance is not a science but an art. This art requires face-to-face evaluation with the family and is the reason to seek treatment advice from a professional.

Once a definitive diagnosis of developmental stuttering is made, treatment can begin. The treatment goals of developmental stuttering are twofold: to decrease the amount of stuttering and to decrease the amount of anticipatory anxiety. Treatment of developmental stuttering follows a two-pronged approach because the severity of dysfluency and anticipatory anxiety are not directly related to each other. That is, some individuals who have the most severe forms of stuttering do not have as much anxiety as some with mild forms. In addition, since these components are not directly related, treating one does not ameliorate the other. Therefore, outlining these two treatment goals best prepares the patient to respond to treatment.

Speech Therapy

Speech therapy is devoted to the treatment of speech disorders, and is usually under the guidance of a speech pathologist. Speech pathologists use many different therapeutic approaches to treat developmental stuttering. There are so many approaches that to present each one would be beyond the scope of this book. However, there are some basic tenets and tools of speech therapy, and those will be addressed.

To treat the dysfluency aspect of developmental stuttering, the patient is taught different ways to produce sounds. Teaching fluency may seem like a futile approach to tackle a genetic, brain-based condition. It is not, however, because brain mechanisms can be manipulated, and manipulation can be taught. Manipulation is possible because the brain is a dynamic organ that can be influenced by environmental and psychological experiences.

Brain Plasticity

Brain plasticity is the ability of the brain to change in response to environmental and psychological stimuli. The concept of brain plasticity was first proposed in 1949 by Canadian psychologist Donald Hebb (1904–1985). Hebb observed that rats raised in a stimulating environment performed better in mazes than rats raised in a less stimulating environment.[5] Hebb believed that the superior performance of the rats raised in a more stimulating environment was due to added stimulation causing the brain to remodel itself to perform better. Specifically, Hebb stated that brain modulation occurred at the neuronal level. The tenets of his proposal were that an enriching environment stimulated neurons in the brain, and that stimulated neurons recruit other neurons to join them. Moreover, repeated neuronal stimulation will promote further connections, and thus change the anatomy and function of the brain to perform better.

Subsequent research confirmed that the brain does remodel itself. Environmental and psychological experiences can cause modulation of the brain at the molecular level. The plasticity of the brain gives credence to the neurological power of teaching, and speech pathologists have at their disposal a cache of tools that can be used to manipulate the function of the brain.

One of these tools is to employ specific maneuvers that can temporarily induce fluency in those who stutter. This is an important aspect in the therapy of fluency. Some of these maneuvers are commonly used in treatment, and some are not. Even though all of the maneuvers do not have a direct place in treatment, their existence offers encouragement to those who stutter.

Maneuvers that Can Induce Fluency

Nine vastly different and seemingly conflicting maneuvers can temporarily induce fluency (Table 4.1). It is not known exactly why these maneuvers work, but the majority of them seem to be connected in one way or another to hearing.

People who stutter can sing with complete fluency. It is postulated that singing is a right brain phenomenon and incorporates other brain circuits than the ones used in speech, which is primarily mediated by areas in the left cerebral hemisphere. This may be the underlying mechanism for the fluency provided by singing. Along with singing, impersonating another's voice evokes fluency. James Earl Jones, the voice of "This is CNN," does not stutter when he performs his famous voiceover; neither does he stutter when he acts. The reason being is that he is using his skills as an actor to impersonate a voice. However, when Jones speaks in his natural voice, he stutters occasionally. In the 1996 film, A Family Thing, he reveals his stutter.

Table 4.1 Maneuvers that can Induce Fluency
Adaptation
Auditory masking
Choral speech
Delayed auditory feedback
Impersonating another's voice
Singing
Speaking alone
Speaking with a metronome
Whispering

The fluency maneuvers of singing and impersonating another's voice are not typically used in speech therapy. However, it is typical to find that those who stutter enjoy singing and are very good at impersonations.

When those who stutter speak in unison with others, which is termed "choral speech," they become fluent. A common example of choral speech is reciting the pledge of allegiance, and a good way to instill confidence in children during therapy is to ask them how bad they stutter while reciting the pledge at school. Invariably, children will answer that they "don't stutter" at this time. This fluency from choral speech helps children grasp that they can speak without a stutter, especially in front of their peers, and is incorporated in speech therapy.

Along the same lines, speaking with a metronome decreases stuttering. There is a cadence one follows when one speaks in unison with a metronome. If the beat is at a slow rate, fluency improves. It has been proposed that speaking with a metronome is a distraction that decreases the anticipatory anxiety associated with stuttering, and hence the anxiety-fueled exacerbations of stuttering. A metronome is commonly used in speech therapy.

Speaking alone, that is, without an audience, also improves fluency. Speaking in front of an audience exacerbates stuttering because the reactions of the audience can decrease the individual's perception of fluency. Moreover, people who stutter tend to believe they stutter more than they actually do, and this perception fuels anticipatory anxiety.

Fluency can also be induced by "adaptation." Adaptation is the noted improvement in fluency when one repeatedly reads aloud from the same text. For example, a father who reads the same book aloud each night to his children will make fewer mistakes on each successive night. This phenomenon is also observed in stuttering. When people who stutter rehearse their speech, that is, repeated narration, they stutter less and less as they repeat their speech. Adaptation in stuttering may simply be ascribed to the efforts of practice; nonetheless, it has a place in speech therapy.

In contrast to adaptation, where people who stutter become fluent by listening to their own voice, fluency can be induced when people who stutter do not hear themselves talk. For example, people who stutter speak more fluently when they whisper. This effect is more profound when hearing is completely detached from speaking. Auditory masking is a maneuver that completely prevents persons from hearing themselves talk. This is simply accomplished by using loud noise to mask speech. Commonly, white noise is played in a room or in a headset. White noise is an effective masking sound because it contains all the sound frequencies audible to the human ear, and its fluency-inducing properties are used in speech therapy.

The most recently discovered fluency-inducing maneuver is *delayed auditory feedback*. In 1950, Army engineer Bernard Lee was testing the capabilities of a new electronic tape recorder. One of the novelties of the new equipment was the ability to listen to the recording while it was being taped. Lee tested the new tape recorder by taping his own voice. One day, he mistakenly placed the input for his headset in the wrong jack. Lee noticed his mistake when he listened to the words he was speaking, and found that he had developed a stutter.

The newly developed stutter of Lee was not due to a mistake in the machine recording his voice; he truly had developed a stutter. Lee soon found that the jack he had plugged his headset into caused a short delay in sound transmission from the microphone and the tape he was using to record to the headset he was using to listen to his voice. This delay was quite small; only a fifth of second, but the delay caused him to repeat syllables. He published his observation as an artificial stutter induced by "sidetone delay."

The effect of delayed auditory feedback was not exclusive to Lee. Others who spoke fluently had their speech disrupted by the procedure and also developed a stutter. This is the same today, as anyone who listens to their speech a fraction of a second after it has been spoken will stutter, or extend syllables to notable degree. However, delayed auditory feedback does not have the same effect on people who stutter, that is, they do not stutter more when they undergo the procedure. In fact, the delayed auditory feedback has the opposite effect; they become fluent.

The fluency-inducing mechanism of delayed auditory feedback is a highly debated subject in the scientific literature. Some believe that delayed auditory feedback reduces stuttering in those who stutter by slowing down the rate of speech. This is based on the fact that delayed auditory feedback causes some people to prolong syllables in their speech. Another theory is that the auditory system is involved in stuttering and delayed auditory feedback affects an "auditory feedback loop."

An auditory feedback loop is simply a description of the relationship between speech and hearing. Speech and hearing are connected, and the connection can be conceptualized as a loop. People can modify their speech by listening to it and making appropriate changes in pitch, rate, or volume. For example, volume can easily be raised or lowered to fit the conventions of normal conversation. In this case, the volume of speech is recognized by the auditory system, relayed to the speech apparatus, and then the volume is adjusted. In other words, how speech is heard affects how it is spoken.

Some believe that stuttering is due to a dysfunctional auditory feedback loop, and that delayed auditory feedback can interrupt this dysfunction. There is no consensus on what this dysfunction could be, thus the debate in the literature as to the mechanism of action of delayed auditory feedback.

Whatever the means by which delayed auditory feedback works, whether by slowing down the rate of speech or affecting an auditory feedback loop, the maneuver consistently induces fluency. There are many different delayed auditory feedback machines available commercially, and the range of auditory delay varies according to the machine or protocol used. Most protocols utilize a delay ranging from fifty to three hundred milliseconds. These protocols work well, and seventy to ninety percent of those who stutter will have a decrease in frequency of stuttering with the procedure. Even though the effect is temporary, the fluency-inducing power of delayed auditory feedback has made it a prominent force in speech therapy.

Therapies for Anticipatory Anxiety

In addition to the above-mentioned maneuvers incorporated in the treatment of the dysfluency of developmental stuttering, speech therapy is also directed at decreasing anticipatory anxiety. As with therapeutic approaches to decrease dysfluency, there are a multitude of different methods that address anticipatory anxiety.

Speech therapy approaches range from indirect methods such as reducing environmental stressors that could trigger anticipatory anxiety, to direct methods that diminish anticipatory anxiety by the promotion of confidence through repetition and positive feedback. All of these methods have been shown to be effective in treating anticipatory anxiety associated with developmental stuttering.

One of the more common methods is termed *cognitive-behavioral therapy*. This type of therapy is effective in the treatment of many different brain-derived symptoms, and is used in the treatment of developmental stuttering to decrease anxiety as well as to teach fluency. The method shares some concepts with other forms of speech therapy, and to narrow the broad subject of speech therapy to a digestible concept, the focus here is on cognitive-behavioral therapy.

Cognitive-behavioral therapy (CBT) is symptom-based therapy that incorporates cognitive processes and behavioral theory. The cognitive arm of CBT is to address the cognitive aspects, that is, the thoughts and emotions that underlie a symptom or behavior. The behavioral arm of CBT is the use of behavioral modification, that is, the promotion of specific behaviors to decrease a symptom or behavior. In CBT, these two arms are used simultaneously. The focus of CBT is to address cognitive processes that underlie a behavior or symptom while also using behavioral modification to change these processes. The end result is a decrease of the symptom or behavior.

There are many ways clinicians implement CBT, but the overall method is systematic and time-limited. Commonly, a manual is used and homework is assigned from the manual. Homework allows structure, and is a systematic means by which patients can define their thoughts and practice tasks.

A summary of a protocol of CBT I use in my practice that is primarily directed at ameliorating the anticipatory anxiety of developmental stuttering is as follows: During the first few therapy sessions, I explore with patients the thoughts they have when they become worried about their stutter. I have the patients write down statements that characterize this anxiety, with a direction to make them as concise and pure as they can. Examples include: "I want to hide." "Don't let me blow it again." "They all think I am stupid."

These statements are termed "automatic-thoughts." These thoughts represent the perception patients have regarding their anticipatory anxiety and its effect on the situation they are in. After patients have defined their automatic-thoughts, I have them rate on a scale from 1 to 10, how anxious they become when they experience these automatic-thoughts. Commonly, patients report they are very anxious, with scores of 8 to 10, and also tend to acknowledge other emotions such as anger and frustration. After a few sessions, patients become skilled at the recognition of their perceptions when they become anxious, angry, or mad when they stutter.

The next sessions are directed at exploring if patients' automatic-thoughts are justified. Below is an example of this process.

In the course of CBT, a 10-year-old boy named James had automatic-thoughts that embodied an extreme dislike for school. Discussing the thoughts that came to his mind when he would stutter, James would consistently mention that his overriding thought was hate and specifically stated, "I hate school." James' focus on school was not unexpected, as speaking in front of his classmates exacerbated his stuttering. As a homework assignment, I had him make a list of the reasons he did not like school and the reasons he liked school. James brought back his list at the next appointment, and had ignored my instructions. His list contained only reasons he did not like school, which ranged from the poor quality of food at the cafeteria to annoying classmates. James only cited his stuttering once, and his list did not allude to any frustration or anxiety caused by his stuttering.

After reviewing his list, I ended our appointment early and assigned another homework assignment. I asked him to formulate his list into a 500-word composition, and that this composition should include a section on what he liked about school. Children in the fifth grade are accustomed to writing 500-word compositions, and even though James was not enthralled with this task, he would do it.

At the following appointment, I read the composition, and asked him if he was, indeed, the author. While the composition was completed as assigned and included his reasons that he did not like school and a statement that he enjoyed "field trips and reading," my suspicion was that it was a forgery. The composition was too good to be authored by a child who hated school. Other than the salutation of "peace out," the composition was one of scholarship. The author's handwriting was impeccable, the vocabulary was plush, and the commas were in all the right places.

I asked James if his mother had written the composition for him. Without a stutter, James answered that he wrote the composition and proclaimed that his mother would vouch for him. James brought his mother into the office, and she assured me that James was, without a doubt, the author. In addition, James insisted that he was not a "cheater;" however, he believed some of his classmates could be labeled as such.

After further clarification that James was undeniably the author, James and I spent time discussing why he was a gifted writer. The consensus reached in discussion was that he was a skilled writer because he performed well in school. Moreover, he liked that he was an accomplished student. After some deliberation, James admitted that he didn't hate school and that this automatic-thought was not a true reflection of how he really felt.

After patients have evaluated whether their automatic-thoughts are justified, I spend the last sessions of CBT promoting automatic-thoughts that are positive. This last stage of CBT incorporates behavioral modification to promote these positive automatic-thoughts. In James' case, these thoughts were that he liked school and was smart, and these thoughts were promoted via encouragement and rehearsal of his public speaking. In short, this last stage is spent teaching a new means by which to think about a situation and this learning is based on repetition.

> James and I spent our final sessions rehearsing public speaking. Public speaking exacerbated his stutter, and this was directly related to his anxiety. Alleviating his anticipatory anxiety was the focus of our therapy, and our approach entailed practice.
>
> As final homework assignments, I had James write other compositions on subjects in which he was interested, such as skateboarding. He read his reports to an audience consisting of his mother, administrative staff, and myself. James occasionally stuttered during these presentations, and was visibly frustrated.
>
> When he stuttered, we calmly waited for him to continue and ignored his attempts to quit. This patience was, in part, due to my directions and, in part, due to the subject matter. It was helpful to learn that it is poor form to "shank a vert" while skateboarding, and the audience appreciated this guidance.
>
> After James presented his material, we spent time discussing his presentations and focused on the times he stuttered. To reinforce positive automatic-thoughts, I reiterated that when he speaks, the audience is listening to the content of his words and is less concerned with the form—especially in his case, as smart people usually have something interesting to say. After several sessions, James' fluency improved during his presentations. In addition, he was more fluent at school. James' improved fluency was the direct result of a decrease in his anticipatory anxiety, and he was able to do this because he had modified his thoughts.

There are many different ways to practice CBT other than what was presented in the case study above. The methods vary, but the central tenet is that by modifying one's thinking—in that irrational thoughts are identified and discounted and positive thoughts are promoted—behaviors can change. Outcome studies have proved CBT to be successful in treating developmental stuttering, as well as other brain-based conditions. The scientific explanation for this phenomenon is ascribed to brain plasticity, and CBT has been shown to cause observable changes in the brain.

The landmark study of CBT and brain plasticity was performed by Lewis Baxter and his colleagues from the Department of Psychiatry at the University of California, Los Angeles. In 1992, Baxter and his colleagues presented findings from a PET study they had done to measure brain activity in patients who had been treated for anxiety. One cohort was treated with medications, and another cohort was treated with CBT.

The majority of patients responded to treatment, and the response rate was approximately the same for both groups. When post-treatment PET scans were performed, the medication cohort of patients had the same changes in brain activity as the cohort whom received CBT as treatment. These results reveal that the treatment of anxiety causes changes in brain activity. Moreover, the results show that therapy can produce brain function changes similar to brain-specific medication. This result is a reflection of brain plasticity and the power of therapy.

The Efficacy of Speech Therapy

Speech therapy—verbal instruction and systematic practice—can not only induce fluency, but also actually influence the function of the brain in a demonstrable way—that is, via brain imaging. Recent neuroimaging results have shown what clinicians have known for some time now: With instruction, one can think oneself to speak fluently. Now knowing how speech therapy works—that is, by modulating brain function—the question arises: How well does it work?

Speech therapy works quite well. In review of the over 100 studies of the efficacy of speech therapy, 60 to 80 percents of adults with developmental stuttering have substantial improvement with speech therapy, no matter what specific nuances or maneuvers are incorporated into the therapy. That adults have this high response to treatment is important, as it cannot be attributed to spontaneous recovery.

Developmental stuttering has an 80 percent spontaneous recovery rate. This recovery primarily occurs in childhood, and about 90 percent of the children who spontaneously recover will do so within five years of the onset of developmental stuttering. So, most adults who benefit from speech therapy do so because of the therapy.

In addition, study of speech therapy shows that it is of most benefit in younger patients. Younger patients, that is, preschool patients who have just begun to stutter, appear to respond to therapy in a shorter period of time, and do so with more ease. However, this observation needs to be tempered with the fact that the preschool and elementary school population is the cohort that has the highest rate of spontaneous recovery. As such, early treatment of the youngest children with developmental stuttering is a highly debated subject in the scientific literature. Proponents of early intervention argue that speech therapy is most successful in young children and therefore should be started as soon as possible. Other clinicians believe that treating every child who stutters is wasteful as it addresses children who would recover on their own and diverts resources from those who would benefit. Both sides of this debate have valid points, and the best way to determine which side is the best is to spend some time with the doctor.

While speech therapy is the mainstay of treatment and has a high success rate, there are ways to directly induce fluency and the decrease anticipatory anxiety at the molecular level. This direct modulation is possible through pharmacological compounds that act in the brain and target brain function. As the role of the brain in developmental stuttering has become better understood and psychopharmacology has become more sophisticated, medicines have assumed a role and are used to successfully treat developmental stuttering.

Medications

Following the understanding that recent breakthroughs in neuroimaging and genetics have provided, psychopharmacology has become effective in the treatment of brain-based disease. Science has advanced to the stage where medicines are developed and prescribed in accordance to the underlying molecular causes of many different diseases of the brain. Depression, Parkinson disease, and schizophrenia are some of the many brain-based illnesses that have benefited from recent advances in psychopharmacology. As developmental stuttering has been discovered to be a brain-based condition, it too is reaping these benefits.

As it stands now, no medications can cure developmental stuttering, but some can significantly reduce its symptoms. This improvement is due to the direct effect of medication on the molecular mechanisms that underlie developmental stuttering, and the two brain-based mechanisms targeted are those associated with fluency and anticipatory anxiety.

Medications that Induce Fluency

Many medications have been used to induce fluency in those who stutter. Most have not been found to be successful. These medications have failed outright or have not shown to be efficacious when subjected to the current standard of scientific scrutiny. This acceptable standard is evaluation by a double-blind, placebo-controlled trial.

A double-blind, placebo-controlled trial is the gold standard for evaluating the efficacy of a medication, as it is designed to eliminate bias from the participants. This bias is negated by the "double-blind" of the trial, in that, neither the patients enrolled in the trial nor the investigators studying the medication know which patients are receiving medication or placebo. This blind is lifted after completion of the trial. Then the investigators can eliminate the placebo response, which is the psychological benefit observed when one knows one is receiving treatment. If the patients in the placebo group show improvement, which is usually the case to some degree, this improvement is subtracted from the response observed in the cohort of patients who received medication.

The scrutiny of the double-blind, placebo-controlled trial has eliminated many different medications that were thought to have some benefit in inducing fluency. However, there are two medications that have passed this evaluation. In addition, there is another medication that has worked well in preliminary studies, and is currently being evaluated in a double-blind, placebo-controlled trial. These three medications share a similar mechanism of action and, in light of what is currently known about brain function in developmental stuttering, their efficacy is understandable.

Haloperidol

Haloperidol (Haldol®) was the first medication that passed double-blind, placebo-controlled scrutiny, and has been the subject of more treatment trials for developmental stuttering than any other medication. Haloperidol is a synthetic compound that was developed by the Belgian physician Paul Janseen in the late 1950s.

Haloperidol works by blocking dopamine receptors in the brain, and specifically targets the dopamine-2 receptor, which is one of the five different dopamine receptors in the brain. By blocking dopamine-2 receptors, haloperidol prevents the binding of dopamine to its receptor in the synaptic cleft. This action decreases dopaminergic transmission between neurons, which is a benefit in treating brain-based diseases associated with increased dopaminergic activity.

There are many different brain-based illnesses and symptoms that are associated with increased dopaminergic activity. In addition to developmental stuttering, Tourette syndrome is associated with increased dopaminergic activity; the reason haloperidol was first used in developmental stuttering was because of its success in treating Tourette syndrome.

By the early 1960s, haloperidol had been found to be an effective treatment for Tourette syndrome and other tic disorders. As Tourette syndrome shares many characteristics with developmental stuttering, physicians began to systematically evaluate haloperidol in the treatment of developmental stuttering. In 1971, P. G. Wells and

M. T. Malcolm from the Royal Southern Hospital, Liverpool, reported their results of the first double-blind, placebo-controlled trial evaluating the use of haloperidol in developmental stuttering. They found that haloperidol was strikingly more effective than placebo in promoting fluency. These results were replicated in other double-blind, placebo-controlled studies throughout the 1970s, and it is an established fact that haloperidol induces fluency in individuals with developmental stuttering.

However, haloperidol is not recommended for developmental stuttering, because its side effects are more troublesome than stuttering. Haloperidol, because it is such a strong blocker of dopamine, causes side effects that resemble Parkinson disease. Parkinson disease is caused by a depletion of dopaminergic neurons, and has symptoms such as tremors, muscle stiffness, slow movements, and gait difficulties. Side effects of medications that resemble Parkinson disease are commonly termed "extrapyramidal side effects" (EPS), as they are mediated by the extrapyramidal motor system found in the basal ganglia. EPS are noted with haloperidol, and have been observed in patients treated with haloperidol for their stuttering. In addition, haloperidol causes akathisia, which is motor restlessness that can range from an urge to move about to actual random movements. EPS and akathisia are side effects that can be treated by the addition of other medications. However, haloperidol—if given over many years—may cause tardive dyskinesia, which is a rare, permanent condition characterized by involuntary movements of the tongue and facial muscles. There is no effective treatment for tardive dyskinesia, and fortunately, it has not been reported in any of the patients who received haloperidol for their stuttering. However, the risk of tardive dyskinesia and the other side effects of haloperidol outweigh the benefits of fluency, and it is not currently recommended for those who stutter.

Even though haloperidol has side effects that limit its use, the study of its effect on brain function stimulated the development of a new generation of medications that retain the efficacy of haloperidol, while decreasing the side effects. These medications have shown promise in the treatment of developmental stuttering, and are termed "serotonin-dopamine antagonists."

Serotonin-Dopamine Antagonists

Serotonin-dopamine antagonists (SDAs) are a class of medications that simultaneously block serotonin and dopamine receptors. Like dopamine, serotonin is a neurotransmitter that is found in the brain. The serotonergic system arises from the brain stem and projects to various areas of the brain. The serotonergic pathways are more complicated than the four discrete pathways noted in the dopaminergic system, and serotonin is found in other areas of the body than the brain. As it is dispersed throughout the body, serotonin plays a role in many different biochemical systems. However as serotonin relates to the SDAs, its blockage provides a major benefit as it significantly decreases the risk of the side effects found with haloperidol while maintaining efficacy.

SDAs have a low incidence of akathisia, EPS, and tardive dyskinesia because they were specifically designed to block the serotonin-2 receptor, more commonly written as an abbreviation of its chemical name, 5HT-2 (5-hydroxytryptamine). The 5HT-2 receptor is one of 17 different types of serotonin receptors that have been identified. The importance of 5HT-2 receptors in drug development first became noted in the 1970s when a medication named clozapine was introduced for schizophrenia. Clozapine worked extremely well for schizophrenia. Moreover, it did not have any of the typical above-mentioned side effects noted with haloperidol. Thus, clozapine was termed "atypical." However, clozapine was soon withdrawn from the market, as it is associated with fatal bone marrow toxicity.[6]

The promise of clozapine encouraged researchers to explore why clozapine was atypical, and to develop medications that were clozapine-like, but without toxicity. These investigations revealed that clozapine was atypical because it strongly blocks 5HT-2 receptors. Soon after, medications were developed that were atypical, nontoxic, and efficacious. In the 1990s, the SDAs emerged as a new generation of medications for brain-based conditions.

Currently, four SDAs are available: risperidone (Risperdal®); olanzapine (Zyprexa®); quetiapine (Seroquel®); and ziprasidone (Geodon®). There are several others in advanced stages of clinical trials, and these medications may be approved soon. Of the available SDAs, risperidone and olanzapine have been successfully used to induce fluency in those who stutter.

The first of the SDAs to enter the market was *risperidone*. Risperidone was introduced in the United States in 1994, and has been the most studied of the SDAs. Risperidone is a potent blocker of dopamine-2 and 5HT-2 receptors. As it was designed, risperidone has been observed to be atypical, and has been used successfully in many brain-based conditions.

Risperidone was first used in developmental stuttering in 1997 under the direction of Gerald Maguire from the Department of Psychiatry at the University of California, Irvine. Maguire and his colleagues prescribed low-dose risperidone to four adult patients with developmental stuttering. Over a four-week trial, risperidone increased fluency and did not cause side effects. Maguire himself was one of the patients, as he has stuttered since childhood.

Following the success of this pilot study, and the emergence in the literature of the successful treatment of Tourette syndrome with risperidone, Maguire conducted a double-blind, placebo-controlled trial in 16 adults with developmental stuttering, and presented his results in 2000. As in the pilot study, risperidone significantly induced fluency and was well tolerated by the participants. None of the patients acquired the worrisome side effects observed with haloperidol, such as EPS and akathisia. However, sedation was noted in about a third of the patients. This sedation resolved with a decrease of the risperidone. In addition to sedation, there was another side effect observed in the study that, while quite rare, is associated with risperidone.

One of the female patients reported galactorrhea and amenorrhea. Galactorrhea is the secretion of breast milk and amenorrhea is absence of menstruation. These symptoms are normally observed in women during lactation, which is the period after birth when mothers' breast-feed their child. However, this woman was not breast-feeding, and her symptoms were attributed to the risperidone.

As it effectively blocks dopamine-2 receptors, risperidone inhibits the dopaminergic pathway projecting to the pituitary gland (Fig 3.5), and this can affect the regulation of prolactin secretion. Prolactin induces lactation and ovulation, and its release from the pituitary gland is inhibited by dopamine. Risperidone, via the inhibition of dopamine, can induce prolactin secretion and thus cause these side effects. Fortunately, risperidone rarely causes these side effects and when it does, the side effects resolve with discontinuation of the medication. This was the case with this patient.

Despite the sedation and the one case of transient lactation, risperidone was well tolerated by the patients and was significantly superior to placebo in inducing fluency. Risperidone passed the scrutiny of the double-blind, placebo-controlled trial, and along with haloperidol is the only medication to do so.

As it stands now, risperidone is considered a promising medication for developmental stuttering. To gain widespread acceptance, further investigations are required to replicate the results. This is a time-consuming process; however, in the next few years there should be more data on the effects of risperidone in those who stutter.

Olanzapine was the second SDA to pass clinical trials, and was approved for use in late 1996. Olanzapine blocks a number of different receptors with a varying degree of strength, but its mechanism of action is related to its ability to bind dopamine receptors and 5HT-2 receptors. Like risperidone, olanzapine is associated with a low risk of akathisia, EPS, and tardive dyskinesia. Unlike risperidone, and following the observation that the individual members of SDAs differ slightly in their respected side effect profile, olanzapine is not associated with increased prolactin secretion. However, olanzapine is associated with sedation and weight gain. In addition, olanzapine—possibly because of its side effect of weight gain—must be used with caution with diabetics, as it is associated with an increase in blood sugar in these patients.

Olanzapine was first used in developmental stuttering in 1998, and I was involved in these first trials. It was somewhat by happenstance that I became involved in this research. In 1998, while a psychiatry resident at the University of California, Irvine, I was involved with the development of a protocol for the treatment of pediatric delirium.

Delirium is a common brain-based condition characterized by acute, transient confusion that is symptomatically treated with medicines that block dopamine. Delirium is most susceptible in the physically ill, and thus is commonly found in hospitalized patients. The consequences of delirium can be quite harmful to these patients, as in a state of confusion they may injure themselves. For example, it is common for delirious patients to pull out catheters or other monitoring equipment. Moreover, patients become quite frightened when delirious.

As the SDAs had recently been introduced, I collaborated with Lawrence Budner at the Children's Hospital of Orange County (CHOC) to investigate the possible use of SDAs in delirious children. At this time, Budner was the Chief of Child and Adolescent Psychiatry at CHOC, and since CHOC is a tertiary hospital that cares for children with severe illnesses, such as leukemia, delirium is common. Through an extensive review of medical literature, we devised a protocol that incorporated risperidone and olanzapine. We then used our protocol at CHOC. The protocol was helpful, and we eventually published an article about our experience.

About this same time, Maguire was looking into the possible use of olanzapine in developmental stuttering. His inquiry was prompted by the successful observations noted with the use of risperidone. Moreover, he had prescribed the medication to a couple of individuals who were refractory to speech therapy, and it induced fluency. He was curious if it would have the same response in children who stuttered. As I had experience with the use of olanzapine in children, I was asked to help answer this question, and hence my foray into developmental stuttering research and, subsequently, as a treating physician.

In 1999, we presented data from two children, aged 9 and 10, and one adolescent, aged 14, who stuttered. The 9- and 14-year-olds suffered from developmental stuttering, and had not responded well to speech therapy. The third suffered from acquired stuttering secondary to medicine for his AD/HD. All of these children showed a drastic improvement in their fluency with olanzapine, and tolerated the medication well. However, the 14-year-old developed side effects of increased appetite and sedation. These side effects resolved after the dose of the medication was lowered; however, his dysfluency returned. After one month of taking the lower dose, he asked to if he could take his previous dose. We then increased his olanzapine and his fluency returned, yet so did his complaints of increased appetite and sedation. Fortunately, his sedation and appetite returned to normal after three months, while his fluency continued.

In 2000, we presented the other arm of our work, which was the evaluation of olanzapine in four adults who did not respond to speech therapy. The results of this study were similar to our observations in the children and adolescents: Olanzapine significantly increased fluency. However, every one of these patients developed sedation and an increase in appetite. Moreover, in contrast to the adolescent who only complained of an increase in appetite, all of these adults gained weight. The weight gain was moderate, and ranged from two to ten pounds.

Due the promising results in these preliminary studies, olanzapine is currently undergoing the scrutiny of a double-blind, placebo-controlled trial at the University of California, Irvine. If olanzapine passes the test—the results should be out by the time this book is published—it will join risperidone as a promising medicine for developmental stuttering.

Medications that Alleviate Anticipatory Anxiety

The psychopharmacological armament available to treat anxiety is arguably the most powerful in psychiatry. There are many different medications that are successful, and the two most common classes of medications used to alleviate the anticipatory anxiety associated with developmental stuttering are the benzodiazepines and the selective serotonin reuptake inhibitors.

Benzodiazepines

The benzodiazepines are a class of medications first synthesized in the 1950s, and have been safely used in millions of patients since their introduction. There are over twenty different benzodiazepines available, and the most commonly prescribed are alprazolam (Xanax®), clonazepam (Klonopin®), diazepam (Valium®), and lorazepam (Ativan®). Benzodiazepines alleviate anxiety, and prevent seizures and promote muscle relaxation, by binding gamma-amino-butyric acid (GABA) receptors. GABA is the neurotransmitter associated with these receptors and is an inhibitor neurotransmitter, in that it inhibits neuronal firing in neurons it binds to. When benzodiazepines bind to the GABA receptors, they facilitate the inhibitory actions of these receptors. This inhibits neuronal firing at the molecular level, and alleviates anxiety at the clinical level.

Benzodiazepines can alleviate the anticipatory anxiety associated with developmental stuttering within hours, and this effect can last from hours to days depending on which benzodiazepine is used. There are a variety of ways to use benzodiazepines in treating this aspect of developmental stuttering. Benzodiazepines can be prescribed on an as needed basis. This use is helpful for patients who know what types of situations make them anxious. Also, benzodiazepines can be prescribed on a long-term basis. This is common for severe cases of anticipatory anxiety and for prophylaxis.

The side effects of benzodiazepines are quite limited when used as prescribed. Commonly, only sedation and mild impairment of concentration are reported. However, benzodiazepines have addiction potential. This risk is small, and addiction to benzodiazepines is primarily found in the population who abuses other substances. Yet, it is very important to screen patients for abuse before prescribing benzodiazepines. If benzodiazepines are combined with a sedative agent, such as alcohol, this combination can cause a fatal overdose; and steps to prevent such an overdose must be carefully taken by a physician and patient working together. To note, an overdose of a benzodiazepine by itself induces sleep and is not lethal.

Besides the concern with addiction, benzodiazepines have been implicated in cases of acquired stuttering, though this concern is not as significant as the potential for abuse. Acquired stuttering as a result of benzodiazepine use is rare. Moreover, the stuttering resolves when the benzodiazepine is discontinued.

Selective Serotonin Reuptake Inhibitors

The selective serotonin reuptake inhibitors (SSRIs) are a new class of medications that were initially developed for the treatment of depression. Since their introduction in the late 1980s, SSRIs also have been found useful in the treatment of anxiety. There are currently five SSRIs available: citalopram (Celexa®); fluoxetine (Prozac®); fluvoxamine (Luvox®): paroxetine (Paxil®); and sertraline (Zoloft®). Each of these medications has the same mechanism of action, in that all selectively target the serotonergic system.

The SSRIs work by blocking the reuptake of serotonin in the synapse. Serotonergic neurons initiate communication via the release of serotonin in the synapse and end communication by absorbing synaptic serotonin. By blocking serotonin reuptake, the SSRIs immediately increase serotonin in the synapse. This action induces a change in these neurons, and this change—which is not well understood—takes about three to eight weeks to take place. Therefore, the clinical effects of SSRIs are not immediate, but are delayed by about that amount of time.

Even though SSRIs take some time to work, these medications are effective in many different anxiety disorders, and decrease anticipatory anxiety in developmental stuttering. Moreover, SSRIs are not addictive and are safe if there is an overdose. However, the SSRIs are associated with some side effects.

At the start of treatment, it is common for patients to complain of nausea, diarrhea, headache, or even anxiety. For the most part, these side effects are transient and dissipate within a week of treatment. However, SSRIs also can cause sexual side effects such as loss of libido and delayed orgasm. In addition, SSRIs can cause moderate weight loss or gain. These side effects can be treated with medications and by implementing a diet or exercise program.

Also, as observed with the benzodiazepines, there are reports of acquired stuttering with SSRIs. Fortunately, these cases are rare and resolve with discontinuation of the SSRI.

Developmental stuttering is successfully treated. Eighty percent of children spontaneously recover from the condition. Of the twenty percent who continue to stutter as adults, sixty to eighty percent respond to speech therapy. For those refractory to speech therapy, medications can significantly increase fluency and decrease anticipatory anxiety.

Reflecting on two thousand years of futile treatments, this success is quite an accomplishment. Moreover, as science advances, treatment will improve and there will be a cure. The next chapter outlines what steps are being taken to find this cure.

5. Searching for a Cure

The cure for developmental stuttering will arise from a better understanding of the brain processes that mediate the condition. The two most promising investigative fields are neuroimaging and molecular genetics. Functional magnetic resonance imaging (fMRI) is a revolutionary neuroimaging tool that provides the most detailed information on brain functioning; molecular genetics is the study of how genes operate at the molecular level. Researchers worldwide are applying the latest advances in each of these fields in search of a cure.

Functional Magnetic Resonance Imaging

fMRI is the functional application of MRI. Unlike the structural images of MRI, which are obtained from magnetized hydrogen atoms, fMR images are formed from signals produced by magnetized deoxyhemoglobin. Deoxyhemoglobin is a molecule of hemoglobin that has released its oxygen. Active brain cells consume oxygen, and by detecting the changes in amounts of deoxyhemoglobin, fMRI measures brain activity.

fMRI was first developed by Seiji Ogawa and his colleagues at Bell Laboratories in the early 1990s, and advances in the technology have produced images with spatial resolution of about 1 millimeter, which is almost as detailed as structural MRI, and temporal resolution of about 3 seconds, which is about fifteen times better than PET. Thus, fMRI allows detailed mapping of brain function over seconds. The imaging power of fMRI is not the only benefit of the technique. MRI machines are more prevalent than PET and MEG machines and are less expensive to use. In addition, there is no risk of ionizing radiation, which allows obtainment of a greater number of scans on a given individual. These benefits allow more researchers to perform studies on a greater number of individuals, and this accessibility has made fMRI the most widely used functional neuroimaging modality.

However, a problem with applying fMRI in developmental stuttering is that the technology is very sensitive and the head movements that accompany speaking disrupt the localizing power of fMRI. This problem is currently being addressed. Technologies have been recently developed to combine fMRI with MEG and/or EEG to produce maps of brain function with millimeter spatial and millisecond temporal resolution. This integration of modalities will provide superior spatiotemporal resolution, and may overcome the artifact produced by head movements. In addition, Roger Ingham and his colleagues from the Department of Speech and Hearing Sciences at the University of California, Santa Barbara, recently reported the results of a PET study that imaged the brains of adults with developmental stuttering while they imagined they were stuttering. They compared these scans with a control group and with scans of the developmental stuttering group when they stuttered. They found when individuals with developmental stuttering imagine they are stuttering they have the same patterns of brain activity as when they actually stutter. This observation promotes fMRI investigation, as head movements are not produced when imagining.

fMRI studies of developmental stuttering will provide the most detailed view of brain activity. Investigators in Canada, Germany, and the United States are conducting such studies. This technology has the potential to pinpoint the specific brain circuits involved in developmental stuttering, and these findings should enter the medical literature within the next few years.

Molecular Genetics

Molecular genetics is the study of the structure and function of genes. Genes are composed of deoxyribonucleic acid (DNA), which is found in the cell nucleus.

DNA consists of two spirals forming a double helix that are joined together by long sequences of two pairs of bases, guanine-cytosine (CG) and adenosine-thymine (AT). The double helix is held together by weak hydrogen bonds between base pairs. Because pairs form only between A and T and between G and C, the base sequence of each single strand can be deduced from that of its partner.

The sequence of these pairs is how information is coded in the DNA. When the double helix is unwound, the base pairs are exposed and the genetic information encoded in the base pair sequence is available for deciphering.

The genetic code is understood by reading "codons." Codons are bases grouped in triplets. For example, the base sequence "GAA" is a codon. Since codons are triplets that are made up of only four different bases (C, G, A, and T), there are 64 (4^3) possible codons. Those 64 codons form the genetic code.

As an analogy to language, codons can be thought as the code that corresponds to a letter of the biological alphabet. The letters in the biological alphabet are "amino acids." There are 20 different amino acids in humans. However, there are 64 different codons. Therefore, while each codon corresponds to one amino acid, some amino acids have multiple codons. Because of this fact, the genetic code is termed "degenerate."

Once the genetic code is translated to amino acids, the blueprint of life arises to form structures. These structures are "proteins," and accordingly are comprised from a sequence of amino acids. Following the analogy of language, the letters of the biological alphabet are amino acids, while the words of the biological language are proteins. Proteins are molecules that regulate the biochemical processes of life, i.e. they make up the machinery for our development and metabolism. In other words, proteins are the biological words that form the book of who we are.

Molecular Genetic Studies of Developmental Stuttering

There are several different methodologies used in molecular genetic research to identify genes. Presently, there are three research groups looking for the gene or genes involved in developmental stuttering. Each of these groups is using a different methodology.

Dennis Drayna from the National Institute on Deafness and Other Communication Disorders, National Institutes of Health, is heading a study that incorporates a molecular genetic methodology termed "linkage analysis." This type of work entails studying families who have a high incidence of developmental stuttering. Family trees of these individuals are formed, and DNA is extracted from everyone in these families—most commonly from white blood cells.

The linkage analysis aspect of the work is to attempt to "link" known genetic markers that are co-inherited with developmental stuttering. Human genes are distributed on 23 pairs of chromosomes. Genetic markers denote a specific location on a specific chromosome. If a known genetic marker is found to be highly prevalent in family members with developmental stuttering, then it can be deduced that the gene or genes for developmental stuttering may be close to that marker. This estimates a location for a suspected gene. This process is then repeated utilizing markers that are clustered in the suspected area. Eventually, the location of the gene becomes more precise. Then the DNA in the area can be sequenced base pair by base pair to provide the exact nature of the gene. This methodology has proved to be quite successful in identifying genes involved in disease. For example, the gene that causes cystic fibrosis was identified via linkage analysis.

Drayna and his colleagues are currently examining the entire genome for markers that are co-inherited with developmental stuttering. The families in this study are derived from the population at large, and this is one means by which to obtain a cohort to perform linkage analysis. There are other ways, and there is another group of researchers using a different cohort in their quest to find the gene(s) for developmental stuttering.

Nancy Cox and her colleagues from the University of Chicago School of Medicine are using linkage analysis to investigate the DNA derived from a cultural isolate. A cultural isolate is a population that is isolated from the general population. Cultural isolates are usually found in rural areas of the world, and tend to be religious communities. As these communities are isolated, their genes are less diverse than those of the general population. The advantage in performing genetic research in cultural isolates is that variant DNA is more apparent in a community where the collective DNA is similar. As an analogy to this research approach, it is much easier to identify a yellow car in a crowded parking lot if all of the other cars are blue. Cox and her colleagues are utilizing this advantage by studying the Hutterites of rural South Dakota. The Hutterites have a subset in their community that is afflicted with developmental stuttering. In studying this subset, Cox and her colleagues will be better able to sort through the genome looking for a gene or genes that could be specific for developmental stuttering in that population.

Any gene or genes Cox and her colleagues find associated with developmental stuttering may only be specific for developmental stuttering in the Hutterites, and may not apply to the general population. This is a detriment to genetic work involving cultural isolates. Nonetheless, if a gene or genes are found in the Hutterites that are associated with developmental stuttering, it will allow directed study in those particular areas of the genome in the general population. So to complement their work with the Hutterites, Cox and her colleagues have collaborated with Nicoline Ambrose and Ehud Yairi from the University of Illinois at Urbana-Champaign to perform linkage analysis in families from the general population.

The third group searching the genome is headed by Steven Mee and his colleagues from the Department of Psychiatry at the University of California, Irvine. Mee and his colleagues are using a new technology called "DNA microarray." DNA microarray combines the latest in computer and robotic technology with the knowledge provided by the working dictionary of the genome. The basic technique is as follows: Robots attach known sequences of DNA on a glass chip in a precise, orderly arrangement. The chip provides a platform to match known DNA with an unknown sample of DNA. After attachment, the unknown sample of DNA is washed over the chip. The unknown DNA samples bind—G to C and A to T—to a complementary strand if it is located on the chip.

Technology allows reading of which strands bind, and the unknown DNA sample is identified by the binding pattern on the chip.

Since genes are pieces of DNA, genes that have been sequenced—that is, the sequence of base pairs is known—can be placed on these chips. Presently, technology allows thousands of genes to be attached to a single chip. As the technology improves, which is happening quite rapidly, it will be possible to place the entire human genome on a single chip.

The power of DNA microarray is immense. The technology allows screening of thousands of genes—and soon the entire human genome—at the same time. Also, the technique allows researchers to compare thousands of genes between groups of people at the same time. There are many different types of applications that harness the power of DNA microarray, one of which is gene discovery. Mee and his colleagues are presently gathering a cohort of individuals with developmental stuttering and a control group. They will then use DNA microarray to scan the genome of both groups and determine if there are any consistent variations—that is, a gene or genes particular to the developmental stuttering cohort.

Pathway to a Cure

The findings of molecular genetic research can be applied in a variety of beneficial ways. Once the gene(s) is found, and family and twin studies reveal that there is one or several to be found, the protein(s) it codes for will be known. For example, analysis of the Y chromosome may reveal why developmental stuttering affects males more so than females. Possibly a gene that is expressed more in males or a biochemical process that is particular to males can predispose one to stutter. Molecular genetic research will provide answers to this and many other questions and will clarify what causes developmental stuttering at the level of the protein machinery in the body.

This knowledge provides targets for future treatments. The most common treatment at the molecular level is via medication.

However, in the future, gene therapy—where one targets and corrects the actual gene through molecular intervention—may be an option in the treatment of developmental stuttering.

In addition to treatment breakthroughs, identifying the genetic component of developmental stuttering facilitates diagnosis. Children could be screened by a simple blood test, and treatment could be started as prophylaxis. Also, more definitive diagnoses could be made.

The knowledge derived from molecular genetic research will also be applied to findings from neuroimaging studies, and the convergence of these two fields of study appears to be the most likely pathway to a cure. Once the proteins involved in developmental stuttering are identified through genetic analysis, the neurochemical pathways these proteins mediate will be known. These pathways will be examined in light of the activity observed in the living brain, and this will be the point of complete reassembly of the developmental stuttering solution.

I believe this reassembly is not far off. The convergence of the activity presently observed in the living brain and the molecular machinery produced by the genome is happening rapidly. Now it can be proclaimed that developmental stuttering is a genetic, brain-based phenomenon. However, in the not so distant future, developmental stuttering will be an understood genetic, brain-based condition that will be cured.

Appendix A: How to Converse with Children and Adults Who Stutter

Initially it is uncomfortable to speak with someone who stutters, and it is human nature to address the uneasiness. Stuttering is very noticeable, even in its mildest forms, and the pauses that accompany stuttering may be taken as license for the listener to help out. However, while based on good intentions, many "helpful" actions are not helpful and make the person who stutters feel more frustrated than they already are. Below are some helpful hints on what to do and not to do. While these hints will put you and the person you are speaking with more at ease, the most important thing is to be a good listener. As with all meaningful conversation, what is said is more important than how it is said.

1. Maintain eye contact.

This is a normal part of conversation, and is evidence that the listener is paying attention and is interested. If someone is stuttering, the impression of the listener may be that they are making the person uncomfortable and if they look away the person who stutters will feel at ease and speak with fluency. This has the opposite effect, and highlights the frustration of the person who stutters. It is best to be courteous, patient, and follow social convention by maintaining eye contact.

2. Comment on the stuttering.

Individuals who stutter are acutely aware of their dysfluency and well aware of the common reactions of listeners. A listener is usually not a good enough actor to hide his surprise or reaction when hearing stuttering speech. A kind query of the nature of the person's stutter frees the subject from the taboo realm, and puts the person who stutters at ease. People who stutter have been subjected to all types of ridicule, especially if they stutter severely, and addressing one's stutter is not considered insulting. However, speaking about a person's stutter behind his or her back is rude and annoying.

3. Ask if you do not understand what is said.

Sometimes a stutter may be of enough severity to interfere with the comprehension of what is spoken. This is rare, as most dysfluencies can be understood. Pretending you understand, and ascribing the miscommunication to the stutter, is a detriment to communication. More often than not, the person just misspoke, and the stuttering is secondary. By asking, the person who stutters will appreciate that you are actively listening to what he or she is saying.

4. Do not finish off sentences.

People who stutter know what they want to say. The blocking and pauses characteristic of stuttering is only a problem of speech; it is not a problem of thinking and stuttering is not due to a disruption of thoughts. Finishing sentences for those who stutter may appear to be a helpful maneuver to a listener, but it is not. Patience of the listener is polite. Moreover patience is smart, as the listener may not be able to guess the right word.

5. Do not offer "helpful" speaking tips.

By offering unsolicited advice, the listener assumes the role of a clinician and an expert. This is inappropriate even for physicians or speech pathologists. If it is not in the clinician's office, it is not the appropriate time or place.

Appendix B: Sources of Additional Information

This appendix contains a short list of organizations that provide additional information and support for those who stutter. By no means is this list all-inclusive, and is presented as a starting point for those interested in additional information.

Stuttering Foundation for America
3100 Walnut Grove Road, Suite 603, P.O. Box 11749
Memphis, TN 38111-0749
Toll-free hotline (800) 992-9392
www.stuttersfa.org

The Stuttering Foundation of America is a nonprofit charitable organization that supports stuttering research. In addition, they provide free support and educational services to those who stutter.

The National Stuttering Association
5100 East LaPalma Avenue, Suite 208
Anaheim Hills, CA 92807
Toll-free hotline (800) 937-8888
www.nsastutter.org

The National Stuttering Association is the largest self-help organization for people who stutter. There are local chapters that provide workshops and support group meetings.

National Institute on Deafness and Other
Communication Disorders
National Institutes of Health
31 Center Drive, MSC 2320
Bethesda, MD 20892-2320
http://www.nidcd.nih.gov

The National Institute on Deafness and Other Communication Disorders supports and conducts research in the disorders of human communication. The Institute also offers health information for those who stutter and a means by which to participate in research studies.

The Stuttering Home Page, Minnesota State University, Mankato
www.stutteringhomepage.com

The most comprehensive website on stuttering. Contains a vast amount of information; ranging from the latest research findings in stuttering to first-person accounts.

The Stuttering Center of Western Pennsylvania
The University of Pittsburgh
4033 Forbes Tower
Pittsburgh, PA 15260
412-383-6538
www.pitt.edu/~commsci/stuttering_center/scwp_home.htm

The Center is affiliated with the Children's Hospital of Pittsburgh and the Department of Communication Science and Disorders at the University of Pittsburgh. Their website presents the mission of the Center focusing on treatment, research, education, and support for people who stutter. This website includes an exceptional educational section for parents of children who stutter.

Notes

1. "failed to find": Snidecor, "Why the Indian does not stutter," p. 493.

2. "exert very little pressure": Ibid., p. 494.

3. "were embarrassed by members": Zimmermann, "The Indians have many terms for it: stuttering among the Bannock-Shoshoni," p. 316.

4. "attributing stuttering": Ibid., p. 317.

5. Interestingly, to promote a stimulating environment, Hebb raised rats at his home and allowed them to roam about his house.

6. Clozapine was reintroduced in the 1990s, when it was found to be effective in patients who failed to respond to other medications. However, it can only be used with regular blood monitoring.

Glossary

Acquired stuttering Stuttering due to environmental processes on brain function.

Adaptation The improvement in fluency when a person who stutters rehearses his or her speech.

Akathisia Motor restlessness that can range from an urge to move about to actual movements.

Amino acids Molecules that are the building blocks of proteins.

Amygdala An area deep within the brain involved with aggression, anxiety, and memory.

Anticipatory anxiety Anxiety associated with the fear of stuttering.

Arcuate fasciculus A bundle of nerve fibers passing through the temporal, parietal, and frontal lobes that connects Wernicke's area with Broca's area.

Auditory masking A maneuver that induces fluency by preventing those who stutter from hearing themselves speak.

Automatic-thoughts Perceptions a person has about a situation.

Axon The component of a neuron that transmits an electrical impulse from the cell body to its terminals.

Basal ganglia A cluster of neurons deep within the brain involved in the regulation of motor movements: includes the caudate, globus pallidus, and putamen.

Behavioral theory The use of behavioral modification to decrease a behavior or symptom.

Benzodiazepines A class of medications that bind gamma-amino-butyric acid (GABA) receptors.

Blocking A dysfluency noted in developmental stuttering that occurs between words. When the person attempts to speak, no or little sound is emitted.

Brain plasticity The ability of the brain to change in response to environmental and internal stimuli.

Brain stem The area of the brain that connects the spinal cord with the higher areas of the brain.

Broca's area An area of the brain that is necessary for the motor production of speech.

Cerebellum A bilateral structure below the cerebrum involved with muscle tone and balance.

Cerebral cortex The outer layer of the cerebrum that is divided into functional areas, such as, motor, sensory, and auditory cortices.

Cerebrum The largest and most highly developed area of the brain, composed of two hemispheres; regulates sophisticated mental functions, such as the senses, thinking, and movement.

Choral speech Speaking in unison with others. A maneuver that induces fluency in those who stutter.

Cingulate gyrus An area of the brain associated with emotions and motivational behavior.

Codon A series of three bases that define an amino acid.

Cognitive-behavioral therapy (CBT) A symptom-based therapy that incorporates cognitive processes and behavioral theory.

Cognitive processes Thoughts and emotions that underlie a behavior, belief, or symptom.

Concordance A characteristic that is shared among a pair of twins.

Corpus callosum A band of neurons that connects the right and left cerebral hemispheres and allows communication between the two hemispheres.

Developmental stuttering A condition characterized by specific dysfluency that may be accompanied by secondary motor behaviors and anticipatory anxiety.

Delayed auditory feedback A maneuver that evokes fluency in those who stutter, by having an individual hear what he or she is speaking approximately fifty to three hundred milliseconds after he or she has spoken.

Dendrite The component of a neuron that receives electrical impulses.

Deoxyribonucleic acid (DNA) The molecule that encodes genes.

Diagnosogenic theory of stuttering A theory of the cause of developmental stuttering popular in the mid-twentieth century that was based on parental admonishment.

Dizygotic twins Twins who develop from two different fertilized eggs; they share 50 percent of their genes: fraternal twins.

DNA microarray A molecular genetic technique that analyzes thousands of pieces of DNA at the same time.

Dopamine A neurotransmitter in the brain.

Dysfluency An observed disruption in the normal fluency of speech.

Electroencephalography (EEG) A functional neuroimaging technique that measures the direct electrical activity of neurons.

Electron A negatively charged subatomic particle.

Extrapyramidal side effects (EPS) Tremors, muscle stiffness, slow movements, and gait difficulties noted with medications that block dopamine in the basal ganglia.

Fluency A way to characterize speech that is considered to follow normal, socially accepted time patterns and mannerisms.

Frontal lobe One of the four lobes of each cerebral hemisphere. Involved with complex mental activities and voluntary motor movements.

Functional magnetic resonance imaging (fMRI) The functional neuroimaging application of magnetic resonance imaging.

Gamma-amino-butyric acid (GABA) An inhibitory neurotransmitter.

Gene A sequence of codons that codes for protein synthesis.

Gyrus A raised convolution of brain tissue; a fold.

Haloperidol A medication that blocks dopamine-2 receptors.

Hippocampus An area deep within each cerebral hemisphere that is important for fear and memory.

Hypothalamus An area below the thalamus that regulates body temperature, hunger, and the release of hormones from glands.

Interjection A dysfluency noted in developmental stuttering that occurs between words that incorporate nonverbal sounds, such as um, er, or ah.

Limbic system An evolutionarily old area deep within the brain that is associated with emotions and drives.

Linkage analysis A molecular genetic technique used to locate genes.

Magnetic resonance imaging (MRI) An imaging technique that detects anatomical differences via the magnetic resonance of protons.

Magnetoencephalography (MEG) A functional neuroimaging technique that measures magnetic fields produced by neuronal electrical current.

Molecule The smallest particle of a substance that can exist in a free state and retain the characteristics of the substance.

Molecular genetics The study of the structure and function of genes.

Monozygotic twins Twins who develop from a single fertilized egg; they share 100 percent of their genes: identical twins.

Neuron A nerve cell, which is composed of an axon, cell body, and dendrites.

Neurotransmitter A molecule that communicates electrical messages between cells.

Occipital lobe One of the four lobes of each cerebral hemisphere. Involved in the interpretation of visual information.

Olanzapine A medication belonging to the SDA class.

Parietal lobe One of the four lobes of each cerebral hemisphere. Involved in the processing of sensory information and language.

Photon A packet or quantum of electromagnetic energy. Used as a tracer in SPECT.

Pituitary gland A gland located on the underside of the brain. Produces hormones that regulate a number of biochemical processes, such as growth and metabolism.

Planum temporale An area on the surface of the dominant cerebral hemisphere that is implicated in language. Usually noted to have greater cortical area than its nondominant counterpart.

Positron The subatomic antiparticle of the electron. Used as a tracer in PET.

Positron emission tomography (PET) A functional neuroimaging technique that measures brain activity via positron tracers.

Prolactin A hormone secreted by the pituitary gland that is involved in the regulation of lactation and ovulation.

Proteins Biological molecules that form many structures and regulate the biochemical processes of life.

Proton A positively charged subatomic particle.

Psychopharmacology A field of study devoted to the effects of medication on brain function.

Risperidone A medication belonging to the SDA class.

Secondary motor behaviors Involuntary motor movements that may accompany developmental stuttering.

Selective serotonin reuptake inhibitors (SSRIs) A class of medications that block the reuptake of serotonin.

Serotonin A neurotransmitter. Chemical name is 5-hydroxy-tryptamine (5HT).

Serotonin-dopamine antagonists (SDAs) A class of medications that simultaneously block dopamine-2 receptors and 5HT-2 receptors.

Single-photon emission computed tomography (SPECT) A functional neuroimaging technique that measures brain activity via photon tracers.

Speech pathologist A professional who specializes in the diagnosis and treatment of speech disorders.

Stammering The British term for stuttering.

Stress response The stimulation of the body that allows one to perform maximally during a threatening situation.

Stuttering See developmental stuttering.

Sulci A cleft on the surface of the brain.

Synapse The space between neurons where neurotransmitters transmit electrical signals from neuron to neuron.

Tardive dyskinesia A condition associated with long-term use of medications that block dopamine characterized by involuntary movements of the tongue and facial muscles.

Temporal lobe One of the four lobes of each cerebral hemisphere. Involved with memory, hearing, and emotions.

Thalamus The central area of the brain that processes sensory information.

Tourette syndrome A condition of motor and vocal tics that shares some characteristics with developmental stuttering.

Wernicke's area The area of the brain that is the sensory area of speech.

Bibliography

Abwender DA, Trinidad KS, Jones KR, Como PG, Hymes E. Features resembling Tourette's syndrome in developmental stuttering. *Brain and Language* 1998; 62: 455–64.

Ambrose N, Yairi E, Cox N. Early childhood stuttering: genetic aspects. *Journal of Speech and Hearing Research* 1993; 36: 701–06.

Anderson JM, Hughes JD, Gonzalez Rothi LJ, Crucian GP, Heilman KM. Developmental stuttering and Parkinson's disease: the effects of levodopa treatment. *Journal of Neurology, Neurosurgery, and Psychiatry* 1999; 66: 776–78.

Andy OJ, Bhatnagar SC. Thalamic-induced stuttering (surgical observations). *Journal of Speech and Hearing Research* 1991; 34: 796–800.

Baxter LR, Schwartz JM, Bergman KS, Szuba MP, Guze BH, Mazziotta JC, Alazraki A, Selin CE, Ferng HK, Munford P, Phelps ME. Caudate glucose metabolic rate changes with both drug and behavior therapy for obsessive-compulsive disorder. *Archives of General Psychiatry* 1992; 49: 681–89.

Bhatnagar SC, Andy OJ. Alleviation of acquired stuttering with human centremedian thalamic stimulation. *Journal of Neurology, Neurosurgery, and Psychiatry* 1989; 52: 1182–84.

Blood GW. A behavioral-cognitive therapy program for adults who stutter: computers and counseling. *Journal of Communication Disorders* 1995; 28: 165–80.

Bobrick B. *Knotted Tongues: Stuttering in History and the Quest for a Cure.* New York, Kodansha America, Inc. 1996.

Brady JP. The pharmacology of stuttering: a critical review. *The American Journal of Psychiatry* 1991; 148: 1309–16.

Brady JP. Drug-induced stuttering: a review of the literature. *Journal of Clinical Psychopharmacology* 1998; 18: 50–54.

Brady JP, Ali Z. Alprazolam, citalopram, and clomipramine for stuttering. *Journal of Clinical Psychopharmacology* 2000; 20: 287.

Braun AR, Varga M, Stager S, Schulz G, Selbie S, Maisog JM, Carson RE, Ludlow CL. Altered patterns of cerebral activity during speech and language production in developmental stuttering. An H2 (15) O positron emission tomography study. *Brain* 1997; 120: 761–84.

Broca PP. Perte de la parole, ramollissement chronique et destruction partielle du lobe ant_rieur gauche du cerveau *Bulletin de la Soci_t_ Anthropologique* 1861; 2: 235–38. (Translated by Laurence F. Greenberg, M.D.)

Bryngelson B, Rutherford B. A comparative study of laterality of stutterers and nonstutterers. *Journal of Speech Disorders* 1937; 2: 15–16.

Canter G. Observations on neurogenic stuttering: a contribution to differential diagnosis. *British Journal of Disordered Communication* 1961; 6: 139–43.

Coffey BJ, Biederman J, Geller DA, Spencer T, Park KS, Shapiro SJ, Garfield SB. The course of Tourette's disorder: a literature review. *Harvard Review of Psychiatry* 2000; 8: 192–98.

Conture ED. Treatment efficacy: stuttering. *Journal of Speech and Hearing Research* 1996; 39: S18–26.

DeNil LF, Kroll RM, Kapur S, Houle S. A positron emission tomography study of silent and oral single word reading in stuttering and nonstuttering adults. *Journal of Speech, Language, and Hearing Research* 2000; 43: 1038–53.

Diagnostic and Statistical Manual of Mental Disorders, Fourth Edition, Text Revision. Washington, DC, American Psychiatric Association 2000.

Felsenfeld S, Kirk KM, Zhu G, Statham DJ, Neale MC, Martin NG. A study of the genetic and environmental etiology of stuttering in a selected twin sample. *Behavior Genetics* 2000; 30: 359–66.

Fenichel OM. *The Psychoanalytic Theory of Neurosis*. New York: W. W. Norton & Company, Inc., 1945.

Finn P. Establishing the validity of recovery from stuttering without formal treatment. *Journal of Speech and Hearing Research* 1996; 39: 1171–81.

Foundas AL, Bollich AM, Corey DM, Hurley M, and Heilman KM. Anomalous anatomy of speech-language areas in adults with persistent developmental stuttering. *Neurology* 2001; 57: 207–15.

Fox PT, Ingham RJ, Ihgham JC, Hirsch TB, Downs JH, Martin C, Jerabek P, Glass T, Lancaster JL. A PET study of the neural systems of stuttering. *Nature* 1996; 382: 158–61.

Fox PT, Ingham RJ, Ingham JC, Zamarripa F, Xiong J, Lancaster JL. Brain correlates of stuttering and syllable production. A PET performance-correlation analysis. *Brain* 2000; 123: 1985–2004.

Fukawa T, Yoshioka H, Ozawa E, Yoshida S. Difference of susceptibility to delayed auditory feedback between stutters and nonstutters. *Journal of Speech and Hearing Research* 1988; 31: 475–79.

Gabel RM, Colcord RD, Petrosino. A study of the self-talk of adults who do and do not stutter. *Perceptual and Motor Skills* 2001; 92: 835–42.

Garfinkel HA. Why did Moses stammer? and, was Moses left-handed? *Journal of the Royal Society of Medicine* 1995; 88: 256–57.

Gattuso R, Leogata A. Haloperidol in the treatment of stuttering. *La Clinica Otorinolaringoiatrica* 1962; 14: 227–34. (Translated by Laurence F. Greenberg, M.D.)

Grant AC, Biousse V, Cook AA, Newman NJ. Stroke-associated stuttering. *Archives of Neurology* 1999; 56: 624–27.

Guitar B. Historic treatments for stuttering: from pebbles to psychoanalysis. *American Speech Language Hearing Association* 1989; June–July: 71.

Hebb DO. *The Organization of Behavior: A Neuropsychological Theory*. New York: Wiley 1949.

Helm NA, Butler RB, Benson DF. Acquired stuttering. *Neurology* 1978; 28: 1159–65.

Hodges A. *Alan Turing: The Enigma*. New York: Walker and Company, 2000.

Howie PM. Concordance for stuttering in monozygotic and dizygotic twin pairs. *Journal of Speech and Hearing Research* 1981; 24: 317–21.

Ingham RJ, Fox PT, Ingham JC, Zamarripa F, Martin C, Jerabek P, Cotton J. Functional-lesion investigation of developmental stuttering with positron emission tomography. *Journal of Speech and Hearing Research* 1996; 39: 1208–27.

Ingham RJ, Fox PT, Ingham JC, Zamarripa F. Is overt stuttering a prerequisite for the neural activations associated with chronic developmental stuttering? *Brain Language* 2000; 75: 163–94.

Ingham RJ, Moglia RA, Frank P, Ingham JC, Cordes AK. Experimental investigation of the effects of frequency-altered auditory feedback on the speech of adults who stutter. *Journal of Speech and Hearing Research* 1997; 40: 361–72.

Johnson W. A study of the onset and development of stuttering. *Journal of Speech and Hearing Disorders* 1942; 7: 251.

Kalinowski J, Armson J, Roland-Mieszkowski M, Stuart A, Gracco VL. Effects of alterations in auditory feedback and speech rate on stuttering frequency. *Language and Speech* 1993; 36: 1–16.

Kolb B, Whishaw IQ. Brain plasticity and behavior. *Annual Review of Psychology* 1998; 49: 43–64.

Kidd KK, Records MA. Genetic methodologies for the study of speech. In X.O. Breakefield (ed.). *Neurogenetics: Genetic Approaches to the Nervous System*. New York: Elsevier/North Holland, 1979.

Lajonchere C, Nortz M, Finger S. Gilles de la Tourette and the discovery of Tourette syndrome. *Archives of Neurology* 1996; 53: 567–74.

Lavid N, Budner LJ. Review of the pharmacological treatment of delirium in the pediatric population with accompanying protocol. *The Jefferson Journal of Psychiatry* 2000; 15: 25–33.

Lavid N, Franklin DL, Maguire GA. Management of child and adolescent stuttering with olanzapine: three case reports. *Annals of Clinical Psychiatry* 1999; 11: 233–236.

Lee BS. Artificial stutter. *Journal of Speech and Hearing Disorders* 1951; 16: 53–55.

Lee BS. Some effects of sidetone delay. *Journal of the Acoustical Society of America* 1950; 22: 639–40.

Lee BS, McGough WE, Peins M. A new method for stutter therapy. *Folia Phoniatrica* 1973; 25: 186–95.

Maguire GA, Riley GD, Franklin DL, Gottschalk LA. Risperidone for the treatment of stuttering. *Journal of Clinical Psychopharmacology* 2000; 20: 479–82.

Miller S, Watson BC. The relationship between communication attitude, anxiety, and depression in stutterers and nonstutterers. *Journal of Speech and Hearing Research* 1992; 35: 789–98.

Morgagni GB. *The Seat and Causes of Diseases. Book I. Letter XIV.* Translated by Benjamin Alexander, London 1769. 351–53.

Pauls DL, Leckman JF, Cohen DJ. Familial relationship between Gilles de la Tourette's syndrome, attention deficit disorder, learning disabilities, speech disorders, and stuttering. *Journal of the American Academy of Child and Adolescent Psychiatry* 1993; 32: 1044–50.

Pearson VAH. Speech and language therapy: is it effective? *Public Health* 1995; 109: 143–53.

Raichle ME. Behind the scenes of functional brain imaging: a historical and physiological perspective. *Proceedings of the National Academy of Sciences* 1998; 95: 765–72.

Rastatter MP, Stuart A, Kalinowski J. Quantitative electroencephalogram of posterior cortical areas of fluent and stuttering participants during reading with normal and altered auditory feedback. *Perceptual and Motor Skills* 1998; 87: 623–33.

Rieber RW., Wollock J. The historical roots of the theory and therapy of stuttering. *Journal of Communication Disorders* 1977; 10: 3–24.

Robertson MM, Stern JS. Gilles de la Tourette syndrome: symptomatic treatment. *European Child and Adolescent Psychiatry* 2000; 9 Suppl 1: I60–75.

Rosen BR, Buckner RL, Dale AM. Event-related functional MRI: past, present, and future. *Proceedings of the National Academy of Sciences* 1998; 95: 773–80.

Rosenfield DB. Stuttering. *CRC Critical Reviews in Clinical Neurobiology* 1984; 1: 117–39.

Rosenzweig MR, Bennett EL. Psychobiology of plasticity: effects of training and experience on brain and behavior. *Behavioural Brain Research* 1996; 78: 57–65.

Ryan BP, Van Kirk B. The establishment, transfer, and maintenance of fluent speech in 50 stutterers using delayed auditory feedback and operant procedures. *Journal of Speech and Hearing Disorders* 1974; 39: 3–10.

Salmelin R, Schnitzler A, Schmitz F, Jancke L, Witte OW, Freund H-J. Functional organization of the auditory cortex is different in stutterers and fluent speakers. *Neuroreport* 1998; 9: 2225–29.

Salmelin R, Schnitzler A, Schmitz F, Freund H-J. Single word reading in developmental stutterers and fluent speakers. *Brain* 2000; 123: 1184–202.

Sandak R, Fiez JA. Stuttering: a view from neuroimaging. *The Lancet* 2000: 356: 445–46.

Schmoigal S, Ladisich W. EEG investigation in stutterers. *Electroencephalography and Clinical Neurophysiology* 1967; 23: 184–85.

Snidecor JC. Why the Indian does not stutter. *Quarterly Journal of Speech* 1947; 33: 493–95.

Soderberg GA. Delayed auditory feedback and the speech of stutterers: a review of studies. *Journal of Speech and Hearing Disorders* 1969; 34: 20–29.

Stevenson LG. The surgery of stammering, a forgotten enthusiasm of the nineteenth century. *Bulletin of the History of Medicine* 1968; 42: 527–54.

Tapia F. Haldol in the treatment of children with tics and stutterers. *Psychiatric Quarterly* 1969; 43: 647–49.

Timmons BA. Physiological factors related to delayed auditory feedback and stuttering: a review. *Perceptual and Motor Skills* 1982; 55: 1179–89.

Volkow ND, Rosen B, Farde L. Imaging the living human brain: magnetic resonance imaging and positron emission tomography. *Proceedings of the National Academy of Sciences* 1997; 94: 2787–88.

Wells BG, Moore WH. EEG alpha asymmetries in stutterers and non-stutterers: effects of linguistic variables on hemispheric processing and fluency. *Neuropsychologia* 1990; 28: 1295–305.

Wells PG, Malcolm MT. Controlled trial of the treatment of 36 stutterers. *The British Journal of Psychiatry* 1971; 119: 603–04.

Wingate, ME. *Stuttering: A Short History of a Curious Disorder.* Westport, CT: Bergin & Garvey, 1997.

Wood F, Stump D, McKeehan A, Sheldon S, Proctor J. Patterns of regional cerebral blood flow during attempted reading aloud by stutterers both on and off haloperidol medication: evidence for inadequate left frontal activation during stuttering. *Brain Language* 1980; 9: 141–44.

Wu JC, Maguire G, Riley G, Fallon J, LaCasse L, Chin S, Klein E, Tang C, Cadwell S, Lottenberg S. A positron emission tomography [18F] deoxyglucose study of developmental stuttering. *Neuroreport* 1995; 6: 501–05.

Wu JC, Maguire G, Riley G, Lee A, Keator D, Tang C, Fallon J, Najafi A. Increased dopamine activity associated with stuttering. *Neuroreport* 1997; 8: 767–70.

Yairi E, Ambrose N, Cox N. Genetics of stuttering: a critical review. *Journal of Speech and Hearing Research* 1996; 39: 771-84.

Yaruss JS. Evaluating treatment outcomes for adults who stutter. *Journal of Communication Disorders* 2001; 34: 163–82.

Zimmermann G, Liljeblad S, Frank A, Cleeland C. The Indians have many terms for it: stuttering among the Bannock-Shoshoni. *Journal of Speech and Hearing Research* 1983; 26: 315–18.

Zimmermann GN, Knott JR. Slow potentials of the brain related to speech processing in normal speakers and stutterers. *Electroencephalography and Clinical Neurophysiology* 1974; 37: 599–607.

Index

Understanding Health and Sickness Series
Miriam Bloom, Ph.D., General Editor

Also in this series

Addiction • Alzheimer's Disease • Anemia • Asthma • Breast Cancer
Genetics • Childhood Obesity • Chronic Pain • Colon Cancer • Crohn
Disease and Ulcerative Colitis • Cystic Fibrosis • Dental Health •
Depression • Hepatitis • Herpes • Migraine and Other Headaches • Panic
and Other Anxiety Disorders • Sickle Cell Disease